Handbook *of*

Psychiatric Nursing

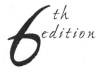

6 th edition

Gail Wiscarz Stuart, PhD, APRN, BC, FAAN
Dean and Professor, College of Nursing
Professor, College of Medicine
Department of Psychiatry and Behavioral Sciences
Medical University of South Carolina
Charleston, South Carolina

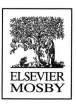

ELSEVIER
MOSBY

ELSEVIER
MOSBY

11830 Westline Industrial Drive
St. Louis, Missouri 63146

HANDBOOK OF PSYCHIATRIC NURSING, SIXTH EDITION
ISBN: 0-323-03502-7

NOTICE

Psychiatric Nursing is an ever-changing field. Standard safety
precautions must be followed, but as new research and clinical
experience broaden our knowledge, changes in treatment and drug
therapy may become necessary or appropriate. Readers are advised
to check the most current product information provided by the
manufacturer of each drug to be administered to verify the
recommended dose, the method and duration of administration,
and contraindications. It is the responsibility of the licensed health
care provider, relying on experience and knowledge of the patient,
to determine dosages and the best treatment for each individual
patient. Neither the Publisher nor the editor assumes any liability
for any injury and/or damage to persons or property arising from this
publication.

Previous editions copyrighted 1988, 1991, 1995, 1998, 2002.

International Standard Book Number: 0-323-03502-7

Senior Editor: Tom Wilhelm
Associate Developmental Editor: Jennifer L. Anderson
Publishing Services Manager: Deborah L. Vogel
Senior Project Manager: Ann E. Rogers
Senior Book Designer: Julia Dummitt
Marketing Manager: Martin Cronin

Printed in United States of America
Last digit is the print number: 9 8 7 6 5 4 3 2 1

Dr. Gail W. Stuart is a dean and tenured professor in the College of Nursing and a professor in the College of Medicine in the Department of Psychiatry and Behavioral Sciences at the Medical University of South Carolina. She received her Bachelor of Science degree in nursing from Georgetown University, her Master of Science degree in psychiatric nursing from the University of Maryland, and her doctorate in behavioral sciences from Johns Hopkins University, School of Hygiene and Public Health. She is Board Certified by the American Credentialing Center as a Clinical Specialist in Adult Psychiatric and Mental Health Nursing, a fellow in the American Academy of Nursing, a member of Sigma Theta Tau, president of the American College of Mental Health Administration, a Distinguished Practitioner in the National Academies of Practice, and a past president of the American Psychiatric Nurses Association. She has also been a van Ameringen fellow at the Beck Institute of Cognitive Therapy and Research and is a visiting professor at King's College, Institute of Psychiatry, at the Maudsley in London.

Dr. Stuart's current position at the Medical University of South Carolina is dean of the College of Nursing. Prior to that appointment she was the director of Doctoral Studies and coordinator of the Psychiatric-Mental Health Graduate Program. She was previously the associate director of the Center for Health Care Research where she worked as a member of an interdisciplinary research team focusing on issues of access, resource utilization, and healthcare delivery systems. She also was the administrator and chief executive officer of the Institute of Psychiatry at the Medical University where she was responsible for all clinical, fiscal, and human operations across the continuum of psychiatric care. Dr.

Stuart has taught in undergraduate, graduate, and doctoral programs in nursing. She serves on numerous academic, pharmaceutical, and government boards and represents nursing on a variety of National Institute of Mental Health policy and research panels. She is a strong advocate for the specialty and is in great demand to speak and consult both nationally and internationally. She is a prolific writer and has published numerous articles, textbooks, and media productions. She has received many awards, including the American Nurses Association Distinguished Contribution to Psychiatric Nursing Award and the Psychiatric Nurse of the Year Award from the American Psychiatric Nurses Association. Dr. Stuart's clinical and research interests involve the study of depression, anxiety disorders, clinical outcomes, and mental health delivery systems.

Running faster, working smarter. It seems like every psychiatric nurse I meet is experiencing the same demands of time, information, and technology. Add to that the increased emphasis placed on evidence-based practice, and one quickly realizes that the need to keep current with these changes is growing, but the time to do so is shrinking. This reality is the reason for this sixth edition of the *Handbook of Psychiatric Nursing*. This new edition has a sharpened focus on presenting the most current, relevant, practical, and concise information about psychiatric nursing care. The compact format makes this content easily accessible to the nurse in the clinical setting. This handbook also serves as an abbreviated complement to the comprehensive text from which it is derived, *Principles and Practice of Psychiatric Nursing*, eighth edition. Thus the reader can learn more in-depth information about any clinical aspect of psychiatric nursing care by accessing the larger textbook, and students can use this handbook as a review and synthesis of content presented in the larger text.

This sixth edition has updated content throughout, information about the latest psychotropic medications, and new tables that summarize the evidence on treatments for the various psychiatric disorders. It also includes information on alternative therapies and, at the end of each chapter, features websites that can be accessed on the Internet, which are related to the chapter's content. In this way readers can stay current with rapidly emerging developments in each clinical area. The text continues to focus on the essentials of psychiatric nursing and is organized around the nursing process, thus providing assistance with conceptualizing, planning, implementing, and documenting nursing care. Nursing treatment plan summaries are included to provide for the clinical application of the nursing process to specific nursing care problems. Both DSM-IV-TR medical and NANDA nursing diagnoses are included, enabling the nurse to maintain a nursing focus while understanding the medical approach as well. Each clinical chapter also includes a patient or family education plan. Whenever possible, tables and boxes are used to present material.

This handbook is divided into two units. **Unit One, Foundations of Practice,** consists of Chapters 1 through 9. This unit is designed to focus on the basic aspects of psychiatric nursing, regardless of the patient care need or the practice setting. Chapter 1 discusses core elements of psychiatric nursing practice. Chapter 2 presents aspects of the therapeutic nurse-patient relationship. Chapter 3 reviews components of a complete biopsychosocial assessment, and Chapter 4 describes nursing and medical diagnoses. Chapter 5 focuses on the often neglected areas of prevention and mental health promotion; Chapter 6 presents aspects of crisis intervention; and Chapter 7 reviews nursing care related to psychiatric rehabilitation and recovery. The legal-ethical issues of care are described in Chapter 8, and Chapter 9 presents the ANA standards of psychiatric-mental health clinical nursing.

Unit Two, Clinical Care, comprises the major content of the book. Chapters 10 through 22 consider nursing approaches to patients with specific nursing care problems, including anxiety, psychophysiological illness, self-concept, disturbances of mood, self-destructive behavior, psychotic and personality disorders, impaired cognition, substance abuse, eating disorders, and variations in sexual responses. The concluding two chapters discuss two specific types of treatment: psychopharmacology and somatic and alternative therapies. These chapters are particularly useful to nurses working in settings that are shifting to a more biological focus on the treatment of mental illness, and they include many explanatory tables and charts.

I want to share with you a personal note of thanks for the wonderful interaction and dialogue you have provided me over the years. Many of you remark how helpful my text has been to you in your clinical work. It is because of such exchanges that I remain committed to providing the information that you need to give the best care possible to the patients and families with whom you work. I dedicate this book to you and all our psychiatric nursing colleagues. Ours is a noble and caring mission. May we carry on with the knowledge, compassion, and commitment our patients so richly deserve.

GAIL WISCARZ STUART

CONTENTS

■ PSYCHIATRIC NURSING DEFINED

Psychiatric nursing is an interpersonal process that strives to promote and maintain patient behavior that contributes to integrated functioning. The patient or client system may be an individual, family, group, organization, or community. The American Nurses Association (2000) defines psychiatric and mental health nursing as a "specialized area of nursing practice employing theories of human behavior as its science and purposeful use of self as its art."

The contemporary practice of psychiatric nursing includes the dimensions of clinical competence, patient-family advocacy, fiscal responsibility, interdisciplinary collaboration, social accountability, and legal-ethical parameters. The psychiatric nurse uses knowledge from the psychosocial and biophysical sciences and theories of personality and human behavior to derive a theoretical framework on which to base nursing practice.

Levels of Performance

The following four major factors help to determine the levels of function and types of activities engaged in by a psychiatric nurse:

1. The nurse practice act of one's state
2. The nurse's qualifications, including education, work experience, and certification status
3. The nurse's practice setting
4. The nurse's degree of personal competence and initiative

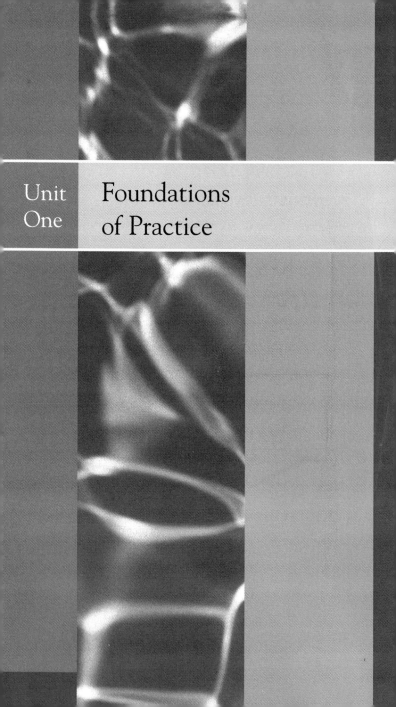

Unit One

Foundations of Practice

There are two levels of psychiatric-mental health clinical nursing practice:

1. A *psychiatric-mental health registered nurse* (RN) is a licensed RN who has demonstrated clinical skills in psychiatric-mental health nursing that exceed those of a new nurse in the field.

2. An *advanced practice registered nurse in psychiatric-mental health* (APRN-PMH) is a licensed RN who has, at a minimum, a master's degree, in-depth knowledge of psychiatric nursing theory, supervised clinical practice, and competence in advanced psychiatric nursing skills. Doctorally prepared psychiatric-mental health nurses in advanced practice have both a master's degree and a doctorate in nursing or a related field.

Levels of Prevention

Psychiatric nursing interventions further include three areas of activity: primary, secondary, and tertiary prevention, as follows:

1. **Primary prevention** is a community concept that involves lowering the **incidence** of illness in a community by altering the causative factors before they have an opportunity to do harm. Primary prevention precedes illness and is applied to a generally healthy population. It includes health promotion and illness prevention.

2. **Secondary prevention** involves reducing the **prevalence** of actual illness by early detection and treatment of health problems.

3. **Tertiary prevention** involves reducing the impairment or **disability** that results from illness.

■ COMPETENT CARING

The three domains of contemporary psychiatric nursing practice are: (1) **direct care,** (2) **communication,** and (3)

management activities. The teaching, coordinating, delegating, and collaborating functions of the nurse's role are expressed within these overlapping domains of practice.

The various activities of psychiatric nurses within each one of these three domains can be further delineated. Box 1-1 lists the range of specific nursing activities that a psychiatric nurse could perform in each area. Although not all nurses participate in all these activities, they do reflect the current nature and scope of competent caring by psychiatric nurses. In addition, psychiatric nurses are able to do the following:

- Make biopsychosocial health assessments that are culturally sensitive.

BOX 1-1

Domains of Psychiatric Nursing Practice

Direct Care Activities

Activity therapy
Advocacy
Aftercare follow-up
Behavioral treatments
Case consultation
Case management
Cognitive treatments
Community assessment
Community-based care
Community education
Complementary interventions
Compliance counseling
Counseling
Crisis intervention
Discharge planning
Environmental change
Environmental safety

BOX **1-1**

Domains of Psychiatric Nursing Practice—cont'd

Direct Care Activities—cont'd

Family interventions
Group work
Health maintenance
Health promotion
Health teaching
High-risk assessment
Holistic interventions
Home health care
Individual counseling
Informed consent acquisition
Intake screening and evaluation
Interpreting diagnostic and laboratory tests
Medication administration
Medication management
Mental health promotion
Mental illness prevention
Milieu therapy
Nutritional counseling
Ordering diagnostic and laboratory tests
Parent education
Patient triage
Physical assessment
Physiological treatments
Play therapy
Prescription of medications
Promotion of self-care activities
Provision of environmental safety
Psychiatric rehabilitation
Psychobiological interventions
Psychoeducation
Psychosocial assessment
Psychotherapy

Continued

BOX **1-1**

Domains of Psychiatric Nursing Practice—cont'd

Direct Care Activities—cont'd

Rehabilitation counseling
Relapse prevention
Research implementation
Social action
Social skills training
Somatic treatments
Stress management
Support of social systems
Telehealth

Communication Activities

Clinical case conferences
Development of treatment plans
Documentation of care
Forensic testimony
Interagency liaison
Peer review
Professional nurse networking
Report preparation
Staff meetings
Transcription of orders
Treatment team meetings
Verbal reports of care

Management Activities

Budgeting and resource allocation
Clinical supervision
Collaboration
Committee participation
Community action
Consultation/liaison
Contract negotiation
Coordination of services
Delegation of assignments

BOX 1-1

Domains of Psychiatric Nursing Practice—cont'd

Management Activities—cont'd

Grant writing
Marketing and public relations
Mediation and conflict resolution
Mentorship
Needs assessment and forecasting
Organizational governance
Outcomes management
Performance evaluations
Policy and procedure development
Practice guidelines formulation
Professional presentations
Program evaluation
Program planning
Publications
Quality improvement activities
Recruitment and retention activities
Regulatory agency activities
Risk management
Software development
Staff scheduling
Staff and student education
Strategic planning
Unit governance
Utilization review

- Design and implement treatment plans for patients and families with complex health problems and comorbid conditions.
- Engage in case management activities, such as organizing, accessing, negotiating, coordinating, and integrating services and benefits for individuals and families.

- Provide a health care map for individuals, families, and groups to guide them to community resources for mental health, including the most appropriate providers, agencies, technologies, and social systems.
- Promote and maintain mental health and manage the effects of mental illness through teaching and counseling.
- Provide care for physically ill patients with psychological problems and psychiatrically ill patients with physical problems.
- Manage and coordinate systems of care integrating the needs of patients, families, staff, and regulators.

Evidence-Based Practice

Accountability for patient care outcomes is a basic responsibility of professional nurses. Central to this accountability is the ability to examine nursing practice patterns, evaluate the nature of the data supporting them, and demonstrate sound clinical decision making in a way that can be empirically supported. This is the essence of evidence-based practice.

Evidence-based practice is the conscientious, explicit, and judicious use of the best evidence from systematic research to make decisions about the care of individual patients. It blends a nurse's clinical expertise with the best available research evidence. Evidence-based practice is also a method of self-directed, career-long learning as the nurse continuously seeks the best possible outcomes for patients through implementing effective interventions based on the most current research evidence. Evidence-based psychiatric nursing practice involves the following series of activities (Figure 1-1): (1) defining the clinical question; (2) finding the evidence; (3) analyzing the evidence; (4) using the evidence; and (5) evaluating the outcomes.

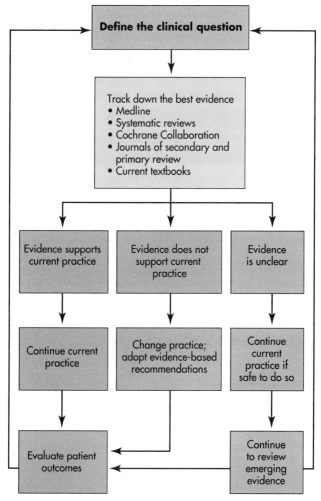

Figure 1-1 Developing evidence-based care.

Outcome Evaluation

Psychiatric nurses must be able to identify, describe, and measure the effect of the care they provide patients, families, and communities. **Outcomes** are those factors that affect the patient and family while they are involved in the health care system, including health status, functional status, quality of life, presence or absence of illness, type of coping response, and satisfaction with treatment. Outcome evaluation can focus on a clinical condition, an intervention, or the care-giving process. The variety of outcomes that can be examined include clinical results, functional improvement, patient and family satisfaction, and financial indicators related to the provision of psychiatric care (Box 1-2).

BOX **1-2**

Categories of Outcome Indicators

Clinical Outcome Indicators

High-risk behaviors
Symptomatology
Coping responses
Relapse
Recurrence
Readmission
Number of treatment episodes
Medical complications
Incidence reports
Mortality

Functional Outcome Indicators

Functional status
Social interaction

BOX **1-2**

Categories of Outcome Indicators—cont'd

Functional Outcome Indicators—cont'd
Activities of daily living
Occupational abilities
Quality of life
Family relationships
Housing arrangements

Satisfaction Outcome Indicators
Patient and family satisfaction with
    Outcomes
    Providers
    Delivery system
    Caregiving process
    Organization

Financial Outcome Indicators
Cost per treatment episode
Revenue per treatment episode
Length of inpatient stay
Use of health care resources
Costs related to disability

Critically evaluating the outcomes of psychiatric nursing activities is a task for every psychiatric nurse regardless of role, qualifications, or practice setting. Psychiatric nurse clinicians, educators, administrators, and researchers all must assume responsibility for answering the question, "What difference does psychiatric nursing care make?"

Your Internet Connection

American Nurses Association
www.ana.org

American Psychiatric Nurses' Association
www.apna.org

Australian and New Zealand College of Mental Health Nurses
www.anzcmhn.org

Canadian Federation of Mental Health Nurses
www.cfmhn.org

Cochrane Collaboration
www.cochrane.org

International Association of Forensic Nurses
www.forensicnurse.org

International Nurses Society on Addictions
www.intnsa.org

International Society of Psychiatric Nurses
www.ispn-psych.org

2 THERAPEUTIC NURSE-PATIENT RELATIONSHIP

The therapeutic nurse-patient relationship is a mutual learning experience and a corrective emotional experience for the patient. In this relationship, the nurse uses the self and specified clinical techniques in working with the patient to bring about insight and behavioral change.

■ NATURE OF THE RELATIONSHIP

The goals of a therapeutic relationship are directed toward the patient's growth and include the following:

1. Self-realization, self-acceptance, and increased self-respect
2. Clear sense of personal identity and improved personal integration
3. Ability to form intimate, interdependent, interpersonal relationships with a capacity to give and receive love
4. Improved functioning and increased ability to satisfy needs and achieve realistic personal goals

To achieve these goals, various aspects of the patient's life experiences are explored during the course of the relationship. The nurse allows for the patient's expression of perceptions, thoughts, and feelings and relates these to observed and reported actions. Areas of conflict and anxiety are clarified. It is also important for the nurse to identify and maximize the patient's ego strengths and to encourage socialization and family relatedness. Problems of communication are corrected and maladaptive behavior patterns are modified as the patient tests out new patterns of behavior and more adaptive coping mechanisms. Figure 2-1 shows the elements that produce a therapeutic outcome.

Therapeutic Use of Self

The principal helping tool that the psychiatric nurse can use in practice is the self. Thus self-analysis is an essential aspect of therapeutic nursing care. Specific personal qualities needed by the nurse who wants to provide therapeutic care include the following:

1. Self-awareness
2. Clarification of values
3. Exploration of feelings
4. Ability to serve as role model
5. Altruistic motivations
6. Sense of ethics and responsibility

Phases of the Relationship

The four sequential phases of the nurse-patient relationship are (1) preinteraction phase, (2) introductory or orientation phase, (3) working phase, and (4) termination phase. Table 2-1 summarizes the nurse's tasks in each phase of the relationship process.

■ FACILITATIVE COMMUNICATION

Communication theory is relevant to psychiatric nursing practice for three major reasons. First, communication is the vehicle for establishing a therapeutic relationship because it involves conveying information and exchanging thoughts and feelings. Second, communication is the means by which people influence the behavior of others. Therefore communication is critical to the successful outcome of nursing intervention because the nursing process is directed toward promoting adaptive behavioral change. Finally, communi-

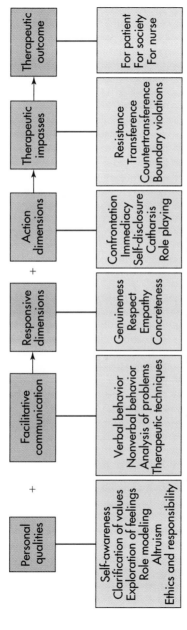

Figure 2-1 Elements affecting the nurse's ability to be therapeutic.

Table 2-1	Nursing Tasks in Each Phase of Therapeutic Relationship
PHASE	**TASK**
Preinteraction	Explore own feelings, fantasies, and fears
	Analyze own professional strengths and limitations
	Gather data about patient when possible
	Plan for first meeting with patient
Introductory or orientation	Determine reason patient sought help
	Establish trust, acceptance, and open communication
	Explore patient's thoughts, feelings, and actions
	Identify patient's problems
	Define goals with patient
	Mutually formulate contract to include names, roles, responsibilities, expectations, purpose, meeting location, time of meetings, conditions for termination, and confidentiality
Working	Explore relevant stressors
	Promote patient's development of insight and use of constructive coping mechanisms
	Discuss and overcome resistance behaviors
Termination	Establish reality of separation
	Review progress of therapy and attainment of goals
	Mutually explore feelings of rejection, loss, sadness, and anger and related behaviors

cation is the relationship itself; without it, a therapeutic nurse-patient relationship is not possible.

Levels of Communication

Verbal communication occurs through the medium of words, spoken or written, and represents a small segment of total human communication. Validation of the meaning of verbal communication between the nurse and patient is essential.

Nonverbal communication involves all five senses and includes everything other than the written or spoken word. The five categories of nonverbal communication are as follows:

1. *Vocal cues* are paralinguistic or extraspeech noises and sounds.
2. *Action cues* are all body movements, including facial expression and posture.
3. *Object cues* are a person's intentional and nonintentional use of objects, such as dress and possessions.
4. *Space* is the physical distance between two people.
5. *Touch* is physical contact between two people and is the most personal nonverbal communication.

The Communication Process

Human communication is a dynamic process that is influenced by the psychological and physiological conditions of the participants. The structural model of communication identifies the following five functional components:

1. *Sender*—originator of the message
2. *Message*—unit of information transmitted from the sender to the receiver
3. *Receiver*—perceiver of the message, whose behavior is influenced by the message
4. *Feedback*—response of the receiver to the sender
5. *Context*—setting in which the communication takes place

If a nurse evaluates the communication process with regard to these five structural elements, specific problems or potential errors can be identified.

Therapeutic Communication Techniques

Two requirements of effective communication are:

1. That it be aimed at preserving the self-respect of both the nurse and the patient

2. That the communication of acceptance and understanding precedes the making of any suggestions or the giving of specific information.

Various methods exist for recording nurse-patient communications, including videotape; sound recording; and verbatim—outline and postinteraction notes. Table 2-2 identifies various therapeutic communication techniques with definitions, examples, therapeutic values, and nontherapeutic threats.

■ DIMENSIONS OF THE RELATIONSHIP

The nurse must acquire certain skills or qualities to initiate and continue a therapeutic relationship. These skills incorporate verbal and nonverbal behavior and the attitudes and feelings behind the nurse's communication. They are broadly divided into responsive and action dimensions, as follows:

1. **Responsive dimensions include genuineness, respect, empathic understanding, and concreteness.** They are crucial in the orientation phase of the relationship to establish trust and open communication. They continue to be useful throughout the working and termination phases and allow the patient to achieve insight.

2. **Action-oriented dimensions include confrontation, immediacy, nurse self-disclosure, emotional catharsis, and role playing.** They must be implemented in the context of warmth, acceptance, and understanding established by the responsive dimensions. They help the therapeutic relationship progress by identifying obstacles to the patient's growth and by underscoring the need for not only internal understanding or insight but also external action and behavioral change.

Table 2-3 summarizes the responsive and action dimensions for therapeutic nurse-patient relationships.

Table 2-2	Therapeutic Communication Techniques			
TECHNIQUE	DEFINITION	EXAMPLE	THERAPEUTIC VALUE	NONTHERAPEUTIC THREAT
Listening	Active process of receiving information and examining one's reaction to messages received	Maintaining eye contact and receptive nonverbal communication	Nonverbally communicates nurse's interest and acceptance to patient	Failure to listen
Broad openings	Encouraging patient to select topic for discussion	"What are you thinking about?"	Indicates acceptance by nurse and value of patient's initiative	Domination of interaction by nurse; rejection of responses
Restating	Repeating to patient the main thought patient has expressed	"You say that your mother left you when you were 5 years old."	Indicates nurse is listening and validates, reinforces, or highlights something patient has said	Lack of validation of nurse's interpretation of message; being judgmental; reassuring; defending

Continued

Table 2-2	Therapeutic Communication Techniques—cont'd			
TECHNIQUE	DEFINITION	EXAMPLE	THERAPEUTIC VALUE	NONTHERAPEUTIC THREAT
Clarification	Attempting to put into words vague ideas or unclear thoughts of patient; asking patient to explain what is meant	"I'm not sure what you mean. Could you tell me that again?"	Helps to clarify patient's feelings, ideas, and perceptions; provides explicit correlation to patient's actions	Failure to probe; assumed understanding
Reflection	Directing patient's ideas, feelings, questions, and content back to patient	"You're feeling tense and anxious, and it's related to a conversation you had with your mother last night?"	Validates nurse's understanding of what patient is saying and indicates empathy, interest, and respect for patient	Stereotyping patient's responses; inappropriate timing and depth of feeling; inappropriate response to patient's cultural experience and educational level

Table 2-2 Therapeutic Communication Techniques—cont'd

TECHNIQUE	DEFINITION	EXAMPLE	THERAPEUTIC VALUE	NONTHERAPEUTIC THREAT
Focusing	Questions or statements that help patient expand on topic of importance	"I think we should talk more about your relationship with your father."	Allows patient to discuss central issues and keeps communication goal directed	Allowing abstractions and generalization; changing topics
Sharing perceptions	Asking patient to verify nurse's understanding of what patient is thinking or feeling	"You're smiling, but I sense that you're really very angry with me."	Conveys nurse's understanding and may clear up confusion	Challenging patient; accepting literal responses; reassuring; testing; defending
Identifying themes	Underlying issues or problems that emerge repeatedly	"I've noticed that in all the relationships you describe, you've been hurt by the man. Do you think this is an underlying issue?"	Allows nurse to best promote patient's exploration and understanding of important problems	Giving advice; reassuring; disapproving

Continued

	Table 2-2	Therapeutic Communication Techniques—cont'd		
TECHNIQUE	**DEFINITION**	**EXAMPLE**	**THERAPEUTIC VALUE**	**NONTHERAPEUTIC THREAT**
Silence	Lack of verbal communication for therapeutic reason	Sitting with patient and nonverbally communicating interest and involvement	Allows patient time to think and gain insights, slows pace of interaction, and encourages patient to initiate conversation while nurse conveys support, understanding, and acceptance	Questioning patient; asking for "why" responses; failure to break nontherapeutic silence
Humor	Discharge of energy through comic enjoyment of the imperfect	"That gives a whole new meaning to the word nervous," said with shared kidding	Can promote insight by making conscious repressed topics; can resolve paradoxes, temper aggression, and reveal new options; is a socially acceptable form of sublimation	Indiscriminate use; belittling of patient; screen to avoid nontherapeutic intimacy

Table 2-3	Responsive and Action-Oriented Dimensions for Therapeutic Nurse-Patient Relationships	
DIMENSION	**CHARACTERISTICS**	

Responsive Dimensions

Genuineness	Implies that nurse is an open person who is self-congruent, authentic, and accessible
Respect	Suggests that patient is regarded as a person of worth who is valued and accepted without qualification
Empathic understanding	Viewing patient's world from patient's internal frame of reference, with sensitivity to patient's current feelings and with verbal ability to communicate this understanding in language appropriate to patient
Concreteness	Use of specific terminology rather than abstractions in discussion of patient's feelings, experiences, and behavior

Action-Oriented Dimensions

Confrontation	Nurse's expression of perceived discrepancies in patient's behavior to expand patient's self-awareness
Immediacy	Current nurse-patient interaction in relationship is used to learn about patient's functioning in other interpersonal relationships
Nurse self-disclosure	Nurse reveals information about self and own ideas, values, feelings, and attitudes to facilitate patient's cooperation, learning, catharsis, or support
Emotional catharsis	Patient encouraged to talk about most bothersome aspects of life for therapeutic effect
Role playing	Acting out a particular situation to increase patient's insight into human relations and deepen patient's ability to see a situation from another point of view; also allows patient to experiment with new behavior in a safe environment

▌ THERAPEUTIC IMPASSES

Therapeutic impasses, or blocks in the progress of the nurse-patient relationship, are of three primary types: resistance, transference, and countertransference. They arise for a variety of reasons and may take many different forms, but they all stall the therapeutic relationship. Therefore the nurse should deal with them as soon as possible. These impasses provoke intense feelings in both the nurse and the patient that may range from anxiety and apprehension to frustration, love, or intense anger.

Resistance

Resistance is the patient's attempt to remain unaware of anxiety-producing aspects within the self. It is a natural reluctance to or learned avoidance of verbalizing or even experiencing the troubled aspects of oneself. Ambivalent attitudes toward self-exploration, in which the patient both appreciates and avoids anxiety-producing experiences, are a normal part of the therapeutic process. A primary resistance is often the result of the patient's unwillingness to change when the need for change is recognized. Resistance behaviors are usually displayed by patients during the working phase of the relationship because it contains most of the problem-solving process. Box 2-1 lists forms of resistance displayed by patients.

Transference

Transference is an unconscious response in which the patient experiences feelings and attitudes toward the nurse that were originally associated with significant figures in the patient's early life. The term refers to a group of reactions that attempt to reduce or alleviate anxiety. The outstanding traits defining transference are the inappropriateness of the patient's response in terms of intensity and the maladaptive use of the defense mechanism of displacement. Transference reactions

BOX **2-1**

Forms of Resistance

- Suppression and repression of pertinent information
- Intensification of symptoms
- Self-devaluation and hopeless outlook on the future
- Forced flight into health, in which patient experiences sudden but short-lived recovery
- Intellectual inhibitions, which may be evident when patients say they have nothing on their mind or are unable to think about their problems; break appointments or arrive late for sessions; or are forgetful, silent, or sleepy
- Acting out or irrational behavior
- Superficial talk
- Intellectual insight, in which patient verbalizes self-understanding with correct use of terminology yet continues maladaptive behavior, or use of the defense of intellectualization when no insight exists
- Contempt for normality, which is evident when patient has developed insight but refuses to assume responsibility for change on the grounds that normality is not so appealing
- Transference reactions

---

are harmful to the therapeutic process only if they remain ignored and unexamined by the nurse. The two main types are hostile and dependent reactions.

Countertransference

Countertransference is a therapeutic impasse created by the nurse, not the patient. It refers to a specific emotional response by the nurse to the patient that is inappropriate to the content and context of the therapeutic relationship or inappropriate in its emotional intensity. Countertransference is transference applied to the nurse. The nurse's responses are not justified by reality but rather reflect problems experienced with individuals from the past or specific issues such as authority, assertiveness, or dependence.

Countertransference reactions are usually one of three types: reactions of intense love or caring, reactions of intense hostility or hatred, and reactions of intense anxiety, often in response to a patient's resistance. Box 2-2 presents some forms of countertransference.

BOX **2-2**

Forms of Countertransference Displayed by Nurses

- Difficulty empathizing with patient in certain problem areas
- Feeling depressed during or after session
- Carelessness about implementing the contract, such as being late or running over the allotted time
- Drowsiness during sessions
- Feeling angry or impatient because of patient's unwillingness to change
- Encouraging patient's dependency, praise, or affection
- Arguing with patient or tendency to "push" patient before ready
- Trying to help patient in matters not related to identified nursing goals
- Personal or social involvement with patient
- Dreaming about or preoccupation with patient
- Sexual or aggressive fantasies toward patient
- Recurrent anxiety, unease, or guilt related to patient
- Tendency to focus on only one aspect of information presented by patient or to view it only one way
- Need to defend nursing interventions with patient to others

Boundary Violations

Boundary violations occur when a nurse goes outside the boundaries of the therapeutic relationship and establishes a social, economic, or personal relationship with a patient. As a general rule, whenever the nurse is doing or thinking of doing something special, different, or unusual for a patient, a boundary violation usually is involved. Sexual contact of any kind is never therapeutic and never acceptable within the nurse-patient relationship. Box 2-3 lists examples of possible boundary violations.

Overcoming Therapeutic Impasses

To overcome therapeutic impasses, the nurse must be prepared to be exposed to powerful emotional feelings within the context of the nurse-patient relationship. Initially the nurse

---

BOX 2-3

Possible Boundary Violations Related to Psychiatric Nurses

- Patient takes nurse out to lunch or dinner
- Professional relationship turns into social relationship
- Nurse attends a party at patient's invitation
- Nurse regularly reveals personal information to patient
- Patient introduces nurse to family members, such as son or daughter, for the purpose of a social relationship
- Nurse accepts free gifts from patient's business
- Nurse agrees to meet patient for treatment outside the usual setting without therapeutic justification
- Nurse attends social functions of patient
- Patient gives nurse an expensive gift
- Nurse routinely hugs or has physical contact with patient
- Nurse does business with or purchases services from patient

must have knowledge of the impasses and recognize behaviors that indicate their existence. Then the nurse can clarify and reflect on feeling and content to focus more objectively on what is happening.

The reasons behind the behavior are explored, and either the patient (for resistance and transference reactions) or the nurse (for countertransference reactions and boundary violations) accepts responsibility for the impasse and its negative impact on the therapeutic process. Finally, the goals of the relationship and the patient's needs and problems are reviewed. This should help the nurse reestablish a therapeutic alliance consistent with the process of the nurse-patient relationship.

 Your Internet Connection

Internet Mental Health
www.mentalhealth.com

Knowledge Exchange Network
www.mentalhealth.org

National Institute of Mental Health
www.nimh.nih.gov

National Mental Health Association
www.nmha.org

The practice of contemporary psychiatric nursing requires that the nurse use a model of care that integrates the biological, psychological, and sociocultural aspects of the individual in assessing, planning, and implementing nursing interventions.

■ BIOLOGICAL CONTEXT OF CARE

New tools and techniques help to explain how the brain works and how the brain, mind, and body interact. The psychiatric nurse must have a working knowledge of the normal structure and function of the brain, particularly mental functions, just as the cardiac care nurse must know how the heart works. Psychiatric nurses can then interpret expanding biological information and its potential for effective treatments to consumers of mental health services and to other health care providers, thus further reinforcing the nurse's role as a patient advocate.

Neuroimaging Techniques

Brain imaging techniques allow for direct viewing of the structure and function of the intact, living brain. These techniques not only help in diagnosing some brain disorders but also map the regions of the brain and correlate them with function. They provide pictures of the working brain. Table 3-1 describes some of these important imaging techniques.

Table 3-1	Brain Imaging Techniques	
TECHNIQUE	**HOW IT WORKS**	**WHAT IT IMAGES**
Computed tomography (CT)	Series of radiographs that are computer-constructed into "slices" of the brain that can be stacked by the computer, giving a three-dimensional view	Brain structure
Magnetic resonance imaging (MRI)	Magnetic field surrounding the head induces brain tissues to emit radio waves that are computerized for clear, detailed construction of sectional images of the brain	Brain structure; newer functional MRI (FMRI) techniques show brain activity
Brain electrical activity mapping (BEAM)	CT techniques are used to display data derived from electroencephalographic (EEG) recordings of brain electrical activity that can be sensory-evoked by specific stimuli (e.g., flash of light, sudden sound) or cognitive-evoked by specific mental tasks	Brain activity/function
Positron emission tomography (PET)	Injected radioactive substance travels to the brain and shows up as a bright spot on the scan; different substances are taken up by the brain in different amounts, depending on type of tissue and level of activity	Brain activity/function

Table 3-1	Brain Imaging Techniques—cont'd	
TECHNIQUE	HOW IT WORKS	WHAT IT IMAGES
Single-photon emission computed tomography (SPECT)	Similar to PET, but SPECT uses more stable substances and different detectors to visualize blood flow patterns	Brain activity/ function

Genetics of Mental Illness

The ongoing search for the gene or genes that cause mental illness has been difficult and inconclusive to date. The complexity of human emotions and behavior is most likely governed by a variety of genes and their interplay with each other, environmental factors, personality, and life experiences.

There are several proposed uses of genetics in psychiatry. These include the following:

- *New drugs* will target molecular regulators of gene expression that control neuroproteins and neuroenzymes in brain regions shown to be abnormal in a particular psychiatric illness.
- *Gene therapy*, the introduction of genes into existing cells to prevent or cure disease, may one day be commonplace for the treatment of psychiatric illness. Studies using "candidate genes" (cloned human genes that are functionally related to the disease of interest) are used in research procedures in the laboratory and are becoming more available for psychiatric research.

Circadian Rhythms

Recent biological research has suggested that body rhythms are governed by internal circadian pacemakers located in specific areas of the brain and that they are subject to change by specific external cues. Circadian rhythm is like a network of internal clocks that time and coordinate events within the body according to an approximate 24-hour cycle. These rhythms affect every aspect of health and well-being, including lifestyle, sleep, moods, eating, drinking, fertility, and illness. Research suggests that one of the most important internal timekeepers is located in the hypothalamus of the brain.

Psychoneuroimmunology

Psychoneuroimmunology is a field that explores the interactions among the central nervous system, the endocrine system, and the immune system; the impact of behavior/stress on these interactions; and how psychological and pharmacological interventions may modulate these interactions. Although the evidence is compelling that psychosocial stressors can temporarily impair the immune response and thus contribute to the development of a variety of illnesses, the role for autoimmunity in the major psychiatric illnesses is unclear. Efforts to relate specific stressors to specific diseases have not generally been successful, but stress is recognized as a potential key to understanding the development and course of many illnesses.

Biological Assessment of the Psychiatric Patient

Psychiatric nurses should include a thorough biological assessment in their evaluation of psychiatric patients. Undiagnosed physical illness can be costly and dangerous if undetected or treated incorrectly. The psychiatric nurse is well suited to screen for the major signs of physical or organic disorders that may complicate a patient's psychiatric status, to identify physical illnesses that may have been overlooked, or to refer a patient for a thorough medical diagnostic work-up if indicated.

A complete health care history of the patient, lifestyle review, physical examination, analysis of laboratory values, and discussion of presenting symptoms and coping responses are essential elements of a baseline assessment (Box 3-1). The nurse should be able to perform a basic physical examination to assess for gross abnormalities and be able to interpret the results of existing, more complex examinations. Appearance, gait, coordination, bilateral strength, tremors and tics, speech, and symptoms such as headaches, blurred vision, dizziness, vomiting, motor weakness, disorientation, confusion, and memory problems should be assessed in detail.

BOX **3-1**

Biological Assessment of the Psychiatric Patient

Health Care History

General health care

Regular and specialty health care provider
Frequency of health care visits
Date of last examination
Any unusual circumstances of birth, including mother's preterm habits and condition
Allergies
Immunizations
Papanicolaou smear and mammogram
Chest x-ray and ECG
TB test

Hospitalizations, surgeries, and medical procedures

When, why indicated, treatments, outcome

Brain impairment

Diagnosed brain problem
Head trauma
Details of accidents or periods of unconsciousness for any reason: blows to the head, electrical shocks, high fevers, seizures, fainting, dizziness, headaches, falls

Continued

BOX **3-1**

Biological Assessment of the Psychiatric Patient—cont'd

Cancer

Full history, particularly consider metastases (lung, breast, melanoma, gastrointestinal tract, and kidney are most likely to metastasize)

Results of treatments (chemotherapy and surgeries)

Lung problems

Details of any condition or event that restricts the flow of air to the lungs for more than 2 minutes or adversely affects oxygen absorption (the brain uses 20% of the oxygen in the body), such as with chronic obstructive pulmonary disease, near drowning, near strangulation, high-altitude oxygen deprivation, and resuscitation events

Cardiac problems

Childhood illnesses such as scarlet fever or rheumatic fever

History of heart attacks, strokes, or hypertension

Arteriosclerotic conditions

Diabetes

Stability of glucose levels

Endocrine disturbances

Thyroid and adrenal function particularly

Menstrual history

Age at occurrence of first menstrual period

Regularity of menstrual periods, impact on lifestyle

Date of last menstrual period, duration

Menopausal history

Assess for premenstrual syndromes

BOX **3-1**

Biological Assessment of the Psychiatric Patient— cont'd

Sexual history

Assess sexual function and activity
Screen for sexual dysfunction
Safe-sex practices and sexually transmitted diseases

Reproductive history

Number of pregnancies, births, children and their ages
Assess birth control methods

Lifestyle

Eating

Details of unusual or unsupervised diets, appetite, weight changes, cravings, and caffeine intake

Medications

Full history of current and past psychiatric medications in self and first-degree relatives
Full history of current use of nonpsychiatric prescription medicines, over-the-counter medicines, and herbal and other alternative remedies

Substance use

Alcohol, drug, caffeine, and tobacco use

Toxins

Overcome by automobile exhaust or natural gas
Exposure to lead, mercury, insecticides, herbicides, solvents, cleaning agents, lawn chemicals
Fetal alcohol syndrome

Occupation (current and past)

Chemicals in the workplace (e.g., pesticides used in farming, solvents used in painting)

Continued

BOX 3-1

Biological Assessment of the Psychiatric Patient—cont'd

Occupation (current and past)—cont'd
Work-related accidents (e.g., construction, mining)
Military experiences
Stressful job circumstances

Injury
Contact sports and sports-related injuries
Exposure to violence or abuse
Rape or molestation

Impact of culture, race, ethnicity, and gender

Physical Examination
Review of physiological systems
Integumentary: skin, nails, hair, and scalp
Head: eyes, ears, nose, mouth, throat, and neck
Breasts
Respiratory
Cardiovascular
Hematolymphatic
Gastrointestinal tract
Urinary tract
Genital
Neurological, soft signs, and cranial nerves
Musculoskeletal
Nutritive
Restorative: sleep and rest
Endocrine
Allergic and immunological
Gait, coordination, and balance

Laboratory Values
Hematology: CBC and sedimentation rate, screen for anemia

BOX 3-1	

Biological Assessment of the Psychiatric Patient—cont'd

Laboratory Values—cont'd

Chemistry, BUN, glucose, thyroid, adrenal, liver and kidney function, etc.
Serology, especially syphilis screen, HIV, hepatitis
Urinalysis, screen for drugs
Stool tests for occult blood

Presenting Symptoms and Coping Responses

Description: nature, frequency, and intensity
Threats to safety of self or others
Functional status
Quality of life
Support system

CBC, *Complete blood cell count;* BUN, *blood urea nitrogen;* HIV, *human immunodeficiency virus.*

Only after a patient has been carefully screened can the nurse determine which of the patient's presenting problems are amenable to psychiatric intervention and which may require a consultant in another specialty.

■ PSYCHOLOGICAL CONTEXT OF CARE

All nurses, regardless of clinical setting, should be proficient in assessing a patient's psychological status and should incorporate the findings into the patient's plan of care. The mental status examination is a cornerstone in the evaluation of any patient with a medical, neurological, or psychiatric disorder that affects thoughts, emotions, or behavior. It is used to detect changes or abnormalities in a person's intellectual functioning, thought content, judgment, mood, and affect and can be used to suggest possible brain lesions. The mental status examination is to psychiatric nursing what the physical examination is to general medical nursing.

Interviewing Skills

The goal-directed patient interview can be facilitated in the following ways:

1. Address the patient by name and introduce yourself and state the purpose of the interview.
2. Demonstrate awareness of and respect for the patient and a sensitivity to the patient's feelings by assuming a warm, empathic approach.
3. Select an environment that provides privacy, physical comfort, and minimal distractions.
4. Listen to what the patient is saying and note underlying themes and omissions.
5. Observe verbal content and nonverbal communication.
6. Allow sufficient time for the interview, and avoid a tense, hurried approach.
7. Monitor your feelings and anxieties in the patient interview.
8. Use secondary sources of information (e.g., medical history, psychological evaluation, social history) as a supplement to, not a substitute for, your clinical impressions and evaluation.

Mental Status Examination

The mental status examination represents a cross section of the patient's psychological life and the sum of the nurse's observations and impressions at that moment. It is not an evaluation of how that patient was in the past or will be in the future. The examination is an evaluation of the patient's current state. The elements of the examination depend on the patient's clinical presentation and the patient's educational and cultural background. It includes observing the patient's behavior and describing it in an objective, nonjudgmental manner. The mental status examination includes information pertaining to the categories listed in Box 3-2.

BOX **3-2**

Categories of the Mental Status Examination

General Description
Appearance
Speech
Motor activity
Interaction during interview

Emotional State
Mood
Affect

Experiences
Perceptions

Thinking
Thought content
Thought process

Sensorium and Cognition
Level of consciousness
Memory
Level of concentration and calculation
Information and intelligence
Judgment
Insight

Appearance. In the mental status examination the nurse notes the patient's general appearance.

Observations. The following physical characteristics of the patient should be included:

- Apparent age
- Manner of dress
- Cleanliness
- Posture
- Unusual gait

- Facial expressions
- Eye contact
- Pupil dilation or constriction
- General state of health and nutrition

♪! NURSE **ALERT**

Dilated pupils are sometimes associated with drug intoxication, whereas pupil constriction may indicate narcotic addiction. Stooped posture is often seen in depressed individuals. Manic patients may dress in colorful or unusual attire.

Speech. Speech is usually described in terms of rate, volume, and characteristics. *Rate* refers to the speed of the patient's speech, and *volume* refers to how loudly a patient talks.

Observations. Speech can be described as follows:

- Rate—rapid or slow
- Volume—loud or soft
- Amount—minimal (paucity), mute, or pressured
- Characteristics—stuttering, slurring of words, or unusual accents

---

♪! NURSE **ALERT**

Speech disturbances are often caused by specific brain disturbances. For example, mumbling may occur in patients with Huntington's chorea, and slurring of speech is common in intoxicated patients. Manic patients often show pressured speech, and depressed patients often have paucity of speech.

Motor Activity. Motor activity refers to the patient's physical movement.

Observations. The nurse should record the following:
- Level of activity—lethargic, tense, restless, or agitated
- Type of activity—tics, grimaces, or tremors
- Unusual gestures or mannerisms—compulsions

 NURSE **ALERT**

Excessive body movement may be associated with anxiety, mania, or stimulant abuse. Minimal body activity may suggest depression, organicity, catatonic schizophrenia, or drug-induced stupor. Tics and grimaces may suggest adverse effects from medications. Repeated motor movements or compulsions may indicate obsessive-compulsive disorder. Repeated picking of lint or dirt off clothing is sometimes associated with delirium or toxic conditions.

Interaction during During the Interview. Interaction describes how the patient relates to the nurse during the interview.

Observations. Has the patient been hostile, uncooperative, irritable, guarded, apathetic, defensive, suspicious, or seductive? The nurse may explore this area by asking, "You seem irritated about something; is that an accurate observation?"

 NURSE **ALERT**

Suspiciousness may be evident in the paranoid or substance-abusing patient. Irritability may suggest an anxiety disorder. Apathy may be associated with depression and seductive behavior with bipolar illness.

Mood. Mood is the patient's self-report of the prevailing emotional state and reflects the patient's life situation.

Observations. Mood can be evaluated by asking a simple, nonleading question such as, "How are you feeling today?" Does the patient report feeling sad, fearful, hopeless, euphoric, or anxious? Asking the patient to rate mood on a scale of 0 to 10 can help provide the nurse with an immediate reading of the patient's mood.

If the potential for suicide is suspected, it is essential that the nurse inquire directly regarding the patient's thoughts about self-destruction. Suicidal and homicidal thoughts must be addressed directly. To judge a patient's suicidal or homicidal risk, the nurse should assess the patient's plans, ability to carry out those plans (e.g., availability of guns), attitude about death, and available support systems.

ᘯ NURSE **ALERT**

Most people with depression describe feeling hopeless, and 25% of those with depression have suicidal ideation. Suicidal ideation is also common in patients with anxiety disorders and schizophrenia. Elation is most common in those with mania.

Affect. Affect is the patient's prevailing emotional tone as observed by the nurse during the interview.

Observations. Affect can be described in terms of the following:

- Range
- Duration
- Intensity
- Appropriateness

Does the patient report significant life events without any emotional response, indicating flat affect? Does the patient's response appear restricted or blunted in some way? Does the patient demonstrate great lability in expression by quickly shifting from one affect to another? Is the patient's response incongruent with speech content? For example, does the patient report being persecuted by the police and then laugh?

 NURSE **ALERT**

> Labile affect is often seen in manic patients, and a flat, incongruent affect is often evident in patients with schizophrenia.

Perceptions. The two major types of perceptual problems are hallucinations and illusions. *Hallucinations* are defined as false sensory impressions or experiences. *Illusions* are false perceptions or false responses to a sensory stimulus.

Observations. Hallucinations may occur in any of the five major sensory modalities, as follows:

- Auditory (sound)
- Visual (sight)
- Tactile (touch)
- Gustatory (taste)
- Olfactory (smell)

Command hallucinations are those that tell the person to do something, such as kill him or herself, harm another, or join someone in the afterlife. The nurse might inquire about the patient's perceptions by asking, "Do you ever see or hear things?" or "Do you have strange experiences as you fall asleep or on awakening?"

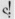 NURSE **ALERT**

> Auditory hallucinations are the most common and suggest schizophrenia. Visual hallucinations suggest organicity. Tactile hallucinations suggest organic mental disorder, cocaine abuse, or delirium tremens.

Thought content. *Thought content* refers to the specific meaning expressed in the patient's communication—the "what" of the patient's thinking.

Observations. Although the patient may talk about a variety of subjects during the interview, the nurse should note several content areas in the mental status examination (Box 3-3). They may be complicated and are often concealed by the patient.

BOX **3-3**

Thought Content Descriptors

Delusion—false belief that is firmly maintained even though it is not shared by others and is contradicted by social reality
  Religious delusion—belief that one is favored by a higher being or is an instrument of that being
  Somatic delusion—belief that one's body or parts of one's body are diseased or distorted
  Grandiose delusion—belief that one possesses greatness or special powers
  Paranoid delusion—excessive or irrational suspiciousness and distrustfulness of others, characterized by systematized delusions that others are "out to get them" or are spying on them
  Thought broadcasting—delusion about thoughts being aired to the outside world
  Thought insertion—delusion that thoughts are placed into the mind by outside people or influences
Depersonalization—feeling of having lost self-identity and that things around the person are different, strange, or unreal
Hypochondriasis—somatic over-concern with and morbid attention to details of body functioning

BOX **3-3**

Thought Content Descriptors—cont'd

Ideas of reference—incorrect interpretation of casual incidents and external events as having direct personal references

Magical thinking—belief that thinking equates with doing; characterized by lack of realistic relationship between cause and effect

Nihilistic ideas—thoughts of nonexistence and hopelessness

Obsession—idea, emotion, or impulse that repetitively and insistently forces itself into consciousness, although it is unwelcome

Phobia—morbid fear associated with extreme anxiety

♩ NURSE **ALERT**

Obsessions and phobias are symptoms associated with anxiety disorders. Delusions, depersonalization, and ideas of reference suggest schizophrenia and other psychotic disorders.

Thought Process. *Thought process* refers to the "how" of the patient's self-expression. A patient's thought process is observed through speech. The patterns or forms of verbalization, rather than the content, are assessed.

Observations. A number of problems can be assessed that involve a patient's thinking (Box 3-4). The nurse can ask various questions to evaluate the patient's thought process. Does the patient's thinking proceed in a systematic, organized, and logical manner? Is the patient's self-expression clear? Is it relatively easy for the patient to move from one topic to another?

BOX **3-4**

Thought Process Descriptors

Circumstantial—thought and speech associated with excessive and unnecessary detail that is usually relevant to a question; an answer is ultimately given

Flight of ideas—overproductive speech characterized by rapid shifting from one topic to another and fragmented ideas

Loose associations—lack of a logical relationship between thoughts and ideas that renders speech and thought inexact, vague, diffuse, and unfocused

Neologisms—new word or words created by patient, often a blend of other words

Perseveration—involuntary, excessive continuation or repetition of a single response, idea, or activity; may apply to speech or movement, but most often verbal

Tangential—similar to circumstantial, but patient never returns to central point and never answers original question

Thought blocking—sudden stopping in the train of thought or in midst of a sentence

Word salad—series of words that seem completely unrelated

♪ NURSE **ALERT**

Circumstantial thinking may be a sign of defensiveness or paranoid thinking. Loose associations and neologisms suggest schizophrenia or other psychotic disorders. Flight of ideas indicates mania. Perseveration is often associated with brain damage and psychotic disorders. Word salad represents the highest level of thought disorganization.

Level of Consciousness. Mental status examinations routinely assess a patient's orientation to the current situation.

Observations. A variety of terms can be used to describe a patient's level of consciousness, such as confused, sedated, or stuporous. In addition, the patient should be questioned regarding orientation to time, place, and person. The nurse usually can determine this by the patient's answers to the following three simple questions:

1. *Person*—What is your name?
2. *Place*—Where are you today (e.g., what city, what particular building)?
3. *Time*—What is today's date?

If the patient answers correctly, the nurse can note "oriented times three." Level of orientation can also be pursued in greater depth, but this area may be confounded by sociocultural factors.

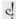 NURSE **ALERT**

Patients with organic mental disorder may give grossly inaccurate answers, with orientation to person remaining intact longer than orientation to time or place. Patients with schizophrenic disorders may say they are someone else or somewhere else or reveal a personalized orientation to the world.

Memory. A mental status examination can provide a quick screen of potential memory problems but not a definitive answer to whether a specific impairment exists. Neuropsychological assessment is required to specify the nature and extent of memory impairment. Memory is broadly defined as the ability to recall past experiences.

Observations. The following areas must be tested:

- *Remote memory*—recall of events, information, and people from the distant past

- *Recent memory*—recall of events, information, and people from the past week or so
- *Immediate memory*—recall of information or data to which a person was just exposed

Recall of remote events involves reviewing information from the patient's history. This part of the evaluation can be woven into the history-taking portion of the nursing assessment. This involves asking the patient questions about time and place of birth, names of schools attended, date of marriage, ages of family members, and so forth. The problem with an evaluation of the patient's remote memory is that the nurse is often unable to tell if the patient is reporting events accurately. Thus the nurse may need to check past records or have family or friends confirm this historical information. Recent memory can be tested by asking the patient to recall the events of the past 24 hours. A reliable informant may be needed to verify this information.

Immediate recall can be tested by asking the patient to repeat a series of numbers either forward or backward within 10 seconds. The nurse should begin with a short series of numbers and proceed to longer lists. Another test of immediate memory is to ask the patient to remember three words (e.g., object, color, address) and then repeat them 15 minutes later in the interview.

ç! NURSE **ALERT**

> Loss of memory occurs with organicity, dissociative disorder, and conversion disorder. Patients with Alzheimer's dementia retain remote memory longer than recent memory. Anxiety and depression can impair immediate retention and recent memory.

Level of Concentration and Calculation. *Concentration* is the patient's ability to pay attention during the course of the interview. *Calculation* is the person's ability to do simple math.

Observations. The nurse should note the patient's level of distractibility. Calculation can be assessed by asking the patient to do the following:

1. Count from 1 to 20 rapidly
2. Do simple calculations, such as 2×3 or $21 + 7$
3. Serially subtract 7 from 100

If patients have difficulty subtracting 7 from 100, they can be asked to subtract 3 from 20 in the same way. Finally, more functional calculation skills can be assessed by asking practical questions such as, "How many nickels are there in $1.35?"

 NURSE **ALERT**

Many psychiatric illnesses impair the ability to concentrate and complete simple calculations. It is particularly important to differentiate among organic mental disorder, anxiety, and depression.

Information and Intelligence. Information and intelligence are controversial areas of assessment, and the nurse should be cautious about judging intelligence after the brief and limited contact typical of the mental status examination. The nurse should also remember that information in this category is highly influenced by sociocultural factors of the nurse, the patient, and the treatment setting.

Observations. The nurse should assess the last grade of school completed, the patient's general fund of knowledge, and the patient's use of vocabulary. It is also critical that the nurse assess the patient's level of literacy. The ability to conceptualize and abstract can be tested by having the patient explain a series of proverbs. The patient can be given an example of a proverb with its interpretation and then asked to explain what several proverbs mean. Frequently used proverbs include the following:

- When it rains, it pours.
- A stitch in time saves nine.

- A rolling stone gathers no moss.
- The proof of the pudding is in the eating.
- People who live in glass houses shouldn't throw stones.
- A bird in the hand is worth two in the bush.

If the patient's educational level is below the eighth grade, asking the patient to list similarities between a series of paired objects may better help the nurse assess the ability to abstract. The following paired objects are frequently used:

- Bicycle and bus
- Apple and pear
- Television and newspaper

A higher-level reply addresses function, whereas a description of structure indicates more concrete thinking. To determine a patient's fund of general knowledge, the nurse can ask the patient to name the last five presidents, the mayor, five large cities, or the occupation of a well-known person.

♂! NURSE **ALERT**

The patient's educational level and any learning disabilities should be carefully evaluated. Mental retardation should be ruled out whenever possible.

Judgment. *Judgment* involves making decisions that are constructive and adaptive. It involves the ability to understand facts and draw conclusions from relationships.

   Observations. Judgment can be evaluated by exploring the patient's involvement in activities, relationships, and vocational choices. For example, is the patient regularly involved in illegal or dangerous activities or frequently engaged in destructive relationships with others? It is also useful to determine if the judgments are deliberate or impulsive. Finally, several hypothetical situations can be presented for the patient to evaluate, such as the following:

1. What would you do if you found a stamped, addressed envelope lying on the ground?

2. How would you find your way out of a forest in the daytime?
3. What would you do if you entered your house and smelled gas?
4. If you won $10,000, what would you do with it?

♩ NURSE **ALERT**

Judgment is impaired in intoxicated patients and in those with organic mental disorders, schizophrenia, psychotic disorders, and borderline or below average IQ. It may also be a problem for manic patients and those with personality disorders.

Insight. *Insight* refers to the patient's understanding of the nature of the illness.

Observations. The nurse must determine if the patient accepts or denies the presence of illness. In addition, the nurse should inquire if the patient blames the problem on someone else or some external factors. Several questions may help to determine the patient's degree of insight. What does the patient think about what the nurse has been told? What does the patient want others, including the nurse, to do about it?

♩ NURSE **ALERT**

Impaired insight is associated with many psychiatric illnesses, including organic mental disorder, psychosis, substance abuse, eating disorders, personality disorders, and borderline or lower IQ. Whether or not a patient sees the need for treatment also critically affects the therapeutic alliance, setting of mutual goals, implementation of the treatment plan, and future adherence to it.

Behavioral Rating Scales

A variety of behavioral rating scales and measurement tools
are available as additional methods of assessment. Rating
scales help clinicians perform the following:

1. Measure the extent of a patient's problems
2. Make an accurate diagnosis
3. Track patient progress over time
4. Document the efficacy of treatment

Frequently used scales include the following:

1. Beck Depression Inventory—self-reporting, 13-item
   scale designed to measure depth of depression and to
   screen depressed patients rapidly
2. Brief Psychiatric Rating Scale (BPRS)—clinician-
   administered, 18-item scale that provides rapid and
   efficient evaluation of treatment response by focusing
   on adult psychopathology
3. Clinical Global Impressions (CGI)—clinician-
   administered, three-item scale measuring severity of
   illness, global improvement, and efficacy of drug
   regimen
4. Hamilton Anxiety Scale (HAM-A)—clinician-
   administered, 14-item scale for patients with a
   diagnosis of anxiety
5. Hamilton Psychiatric Rating Scale for Depression
   (HAM-D)—clinician-administered, 21-item scale for
   assessing severity of an adult patient's depression and
   for showing changes in condition
6. Manic-State Rating Scale—clinician-administered,
   26-item scale that measures manic symptoms,
   including frequency and intensity of behavior
7. Nurses' Observation Scale for Inpatient Evaluation
   (NOSIE)—30-item scale measuring patient behavior
   in adult and geriatric wards, with nursing personnel
   providing measures of patients' strengths and
   pathological states
8. Self-Report Symptom Check List-90 (SCL-90)—self-
   reporting, 90-item scale that presents a list of

problems and complaints and asks the patient how bothersome these problems, if present, have been during the past week

■ SOCIOCULTURAL CONTEXT OF CARE

In each patient interaction the psychiatric nurse should be aware of the broader world in which the patient lives. The nurse should realize that the patient's perception of health and illness, help-seeking behavior, and treatment adherence depends on the individual's unique beliefs, social norms, and cultural values. The culturally sensitive nurse understands the importance of social and cultural forces for the individual, recognizes the uniqueness of these aspects, respects nurse-patient differences, and incorporates sociocultural information into psychiatric nursing care.

Sociocultural Risk Factors

Sociocultural risk factors for psychiatric illness include the following:
1. Age
2. Ethnicity
3. Gender
4. Education
5. Income
6. Belief system

These predisposing factors can significantly increase the potential for developing a psychiatric disorder, decrease the potential for recovery, or both. No one or two of these factors alone can adequately describe the sociocultural context of psychiatric nursing care. Together, however, they provide a sociocultural profile of the patient that is essential to quality psychiatric nursing practice.

Sociocultural Stressors

Lack of awareness of these risk factors and their effect on the individual, along with lack of respect for sociocultural

Table 3-2	Sociocultural Stressors
STRESSOR	**DEFINITION**
Disadvantagement	Lack of socioeconomic resources that are basic to biopsychosocial adaptation
Stereotype	Depersonalized conception of individuals within a group
Intolerance	Unwillingness to accept different opinions or beliefs from people of different backgrounds
Stigma	Attribute or trait deemed by the individual's social environment to be different and diminishing
Prejudice	Preconceived, unfavorable belief about individuals or groups that disregards knowledge, thought, or reason
Discrimination	Differential treatment of individuals or groups not based on actual merit
Racism	Belief that inherent differences among the races determine individual achievement and that one race is superior

differences, can result in inadequate nursing care. Table 3-2 lists some sociocultural stressors that also can hinder the quality of psychiatric care.

Sociocultural Assessment

Assessment of the patient's sociocultural risk factors and stressors greatly enhances the nurse's ability to establish a therapeutic alliance, identify the patient's problems, and develop a psychiatric nursing treatment plan that is accurate, appropriate, and culturally relevant. Box 3-5 presents questions that the nurse might ask regarding each of the risk factors identified.

BOX **3-5**

Questions Related to Sociocultural Risk Factors

Age

What is the patient's current stage of development?

What are the developmental tasks of the patient?

Are those tasks age-appropriate for the patient?

What are the patient's attitudes and beliefs regarding the specific age-group?

With what age-related stressors is the patient currently coping?

What impact does the patient's age have on mental and physical health?

Ethnicity

What is the patient's ethnic background?

What is the patient's ethnic identity?

Is the patient traditional, bicultural, multicultural, or culturally alienated?

What are the patient's attitudes, beliefs, and values regarding the specific ethnic group?

With what ethnic-related stressors is the patient currently coping?

What impact does the person's ethnicity have on mental and physical health?

Gender

What is the patient's gender?

What is the patient's gender identity?

How does the patient define gender-specific roles?

What are the patient's attitudes and beliefs regarding males and females and masculinity and femininity?

With what gender-related stressors is the patient currently coping?

What impact does the person's gender have on mental and physical health?

Continued

BOX **3-5**

Questions Related to Sociocultural Risk Factors—cont'd

Education

What is the patient's educational level?

What were the patient's educational experiences like?

What are the patient's attitudes and beliefs regarding education in general and the patient's own education in particular?

With what education-related stressors is the patient currently coping?

What impact does the patient's education have on mental and physical health?

Income

What is the patient's income?

What is the source of the patient's income?

How does the patient describe the specific income group?

What are the patient's attitudes and beliefs regarding personal socioeconomic status?

With what economic-related stressors is the patient currently coping?

What impact does the patient's income have on mental and physical health?

Belief System

What are the patient's beliefs about health and illness?

What was the patient's religious or spiritual upbringing?

What are the patient's current religious or spiritual beliefs?

Who is the patient's regular health care provider?

With what belief system-related stressors is the patient currently coping?

What impact does the patient's belief system have on mental and physical health?

The psychotherapeutic treatment process also is influenced by the cultural and ethnic context of both the patient and the health care provider. Together the nurse and patient need to agree on the nature of the patient's coping responses, the means for solving problems, and the expected outcomes of treatment.

 Your Internet Connection

American Psychological Association PsychNET
www.apa.org

Dana Brain Web
www.dana.org/brainweb

National Center for Cultural Competence
www.gucchd.georgetown.edu/nccc

ealth-illness and adaptation-maladaptation are distinct concepts. Each exists on a separate continuum. The health-illness continuum derives from a medical worldview. The adaptation-maladaptation continuum derives from a nursing worldview. Thus a person who has a medically diagnosed illness, whether physical or psychiatric, can adapt well to it. In contrast, a person who does not have a medically diagnosed illness may have many maladaptive coping responses. These two continuums reflect how nursing and medical models of practice complement each other.

■ MENTAL HEALTH

The following have been identified as criteria of mental health:
- Positive attitudes toward self
- Growth, development, and self-actualization
- Integration and emotional responsiveness
- Autonomy and self-determination
- Accurate reality perception
- Environmental mastery and social competence

■ MENTAL ILLNESS

One's definition of mental illness is derived from what one believes to be the causative factors. The following hypotheses have been proposed regarding influences on the occurrence of mental illness:

- The *biological hypothesis* proposes anatomical and physiological dysfunctions.
- The *learning hypothesis* proposes maladaptive learned behavioral patterns.
- The *cognitive hypothesis* proposes inaccuracies or deficits in knowledge or awareness.
- The *psychodynamic hypothesis* proposes intrapsychic conflicts and developmental deficits.
- The *environmental hypothesis* proposes stressors and aversive environmental responses.

Box 4-1 presents key facts about mental illness.

BOX **4-1**

Key Facts About Mental Illness

Extent and Severity of the Problem

- The full spectrum of mental disorders affects 22% of the adult population in a given year. This figure refers to all mental disorders and is comparable to rates for physical disorders when similarly broadly defined (e.g., respiratory disorders affect 50% of adults; cardiovascular diseases, 20%).
- Severe mental disorders (i.e., schizophrenia, manic-depressive illness, and severe forms of depression, panic disorder, and obsessive-compulsive disorder) affect 2.8% of the adult population (approximately 5 million people) and account for 25% of all federal disability payments.
- At least 7.5 million children in the United States younger than 18 years of age have a mental health problem severe enough to require treatment.
- Approximately 18 million persons in the United States 18 years of age and older experience problems as a result of alcohol use; 10.6 million of these have alcoholism.

Continued

BOX **4-1**

Key Facts About Mental Illness

Extent and Severity of the Problem—cont'd

- Most alcoholic persons improve through treatment, and evidence suggests that alcoholism treatment is effective in containing costs throughout the health care system and in increasing worker productivity.
- An estimated 23 million people in the United States currently use illicit drugs.

Treatment Efficacy

- How *effective* are treatments for severe mental disorders compared with treatments for physical illness?

Disorder	Treatment Success Rate (%)
Panic	80
Bipolar	80
Major depression	65
Schizophrenia	60
Obsessive-compulsive	60
Cardiovascular treatments	
Atherectomy	52
Angioplasty	41

From National Advisory Mental Health Council: Am J Psychiatry *150:1447, 1993.*

■ NURSING AND MEDICAL DIAGNOSES

Nursing and medical diagnoses may complement each other, but one is not a component of the other. A patient with one specific medical diagnosis may have a number of complementary nursing diagnoses related to the range of health responses. Conversely, a patient may have a specific nursing diagnosis without any identified medical diagnoses.

Nursing Diagnosis

The continuum of **coping responses** is the subject of nursing diagnoses. The continuum may also include actual health problems that lead to a medical diagnosis. A nursing diagnosis is a statement of the patient's nursing problem that includes both the adaptive or maladaptive health response and the contributing stressors.

The North American Nursing Diagnosis Association International (NANDA) has identified, defined, and described a classification system of nursing diagnoses. Box 4-2 lists the NANDA nursing diagnoses.

BOX **4-2**

NANDA-Approved Nursing Diagnoses

Activity intolerance
Activity intolerance, Risk for
Adjustment, Impaired
Airway clearance, Ineffective
Allergy response, Latex
Allergy response, Risk for latex
Anxiety
Anxiety, Death
Aspiration, Risk for
Attachment, Risk for impaired parent/infant/child
Autonomic dysreflexia
Autonomic dysreflexia, Risk for
Body image, Disturbed
Body temperature, Risk for imbalanced
Bowel incontinence
Breastfeeding, Effective
Breastfeeding, Ineffective
Breastfeeding, Interrupted
Breathing pattern, Ineffective
Cardiac output, Decreased
Caregiver role strain
Caregiver role strain, Risk for

From North American Nursing Diagnosis Association: NANDA nursing diagnoses: definitions and classification 2005-2006, *Philadelphia, 2005, NANDA.*   *Continued*

BOX **4-2**

NANDA-Approved Nursing Diagnoses—cont'd

Communication, Impaired verbal
Communication, Readiness for enhanced
Conflict, Decisional
Conflict, Parental role
Confusion, Acute
Confusion, Chronic
Constipation
Constipation, Perceived
Constipation, Risk for
Coping, Ineffective
Coping, Defensive
Coping, Readiness for enhanced
Coping, Ineffective community
Coping, Readiness for enhanced community
Coping, Compromised family
Coping, Disabled family
Coping, Readiness for enhanced family
Death syndrome, Risk for sudden infant
Denial, Ineffective
Dentition, Impaired
Development, Risk for delayed
Diarrhea
Disuse syndrome, Risk for
Diversional activity, Deficient
Energy field disturbance
Environmental interpretation syndrome, Impaired
Failure to thrive, Adult
Falls, Risk for
Family processes: alcoholism, Dysfunctional
Family processes, Interrupted
Family processes, Readiness for enhanced
Fatigue
Fear
Fluid balance, Readiness for enhanced

BOX **4-2**

NANDA-Approved Nursing Diagnoses—cont'd

Fluid volume, Deficient
Fluid volume, Excess
Fluid volume, Risk for deficient
Fluid volume, Risk for imbalanced
Gas exchange, Impaired
Grieving, Anticipatory
Grieving, Dysfunctional
Growth and development, Delayed
Growth, Risk for disproportionate
Health maintenance, Ineffective
Health-seeking behaviors
Home maintenance, Impaired
Hopelessness
Hyperthermia
Hypothermia
Identity, Disturbed personal
Incontinence, Functional urinary
Incontinence, Reflex urinary
Incontinence, Stress urinary
Incontinence, Total urinary
Incontinence, Urge urinary
Incontinence, Risk for urge urinary
Infant behavior, Disorganized
Infant behavior, Risk for disorganized
Infant behavior, Readiness for enhanced organized
Infant feeding pattern, Ineffective
Infection, Risk for
Injury, Risk for
Injury, Risk for perioperative-positioning
Intracranial adaptive capacity, Decreased
Knowledge, Deficient
Knowledge, Readiness for enhanced
Loneliness, Risk for

Continued

BOX **4-2**

NANDA-Approved Nursing Diagnoses—cont'd

Memory, Impaired
Mobility, Impaired bed
Mobility, Impaired physical
Mobility, Impaired wheelchair
Nausea
Neglect, Unilateral
Noncompliance
Nutrition: less than body requirements, Imbalanced
Nutrition: more than body requirements, Imbalanced
Nutrition, Readiness for enhanced
Nutrition: more than body requirements, Risk for
    imbalanced
Oral mucous membrane, Impaired
Pain, Acute
Pain, Chronic
Parenting, Readiness for enhanced
Parenting, Impaired
Parenting, Risk for impaired
Peripheral neurovascular dysfunction, Risk for
Poisoning, Risk for
Post-trauma syndrome
Post-trauma syndrome, Risk for
Powerlessness
Powerlessness, Risk for
Protection, Ineffective
Rape-trauma syndrome
Rape-trauma syndrome: compound reaction
Rape-trauma syndrome: silent reaction
Relocation stress syndrome
Relocation stress syndrome, Risk for
Role performance, Ineffective
Self-care deficit, Bathing/hygiene
Self-care deficit, Dressing/grooming
Self-care deficit, Feeding

BOX **4-2**

NANDA-Approved Nursing Diagnoses—cont'd

Self-care deficit, Toileting
Self-concept, Readiness for enhanced
Self-esteem, Chronic low
Self-esteem, Situational low
Self-esteem, Risk for situational low
Self-mutilation
Self-mutilation, Risk for
Sensory perception, Disturbed
Sexual dysfunction
Sexuality pattern, Ineffective
Skin integrity, Impaired
Skin integrity, Risk for impaired
Sleep deprivation
Sleep pattern, Disturbed
Sleep, Readiness for enhanced
Social interaction, Impaired
Social isolation
Sorrow, Chronic
Spiritual distress
Spiritual distress, Risk for
Spiritual well-being, Readiness for enhanced
Suffocation, Risk for
Suicide, Risk for
Surgical recovery, Delayed
Swallowing, Impaired
Therapeutic regimen management, Effective
Therapeutic regimen management, Ineffective
Therapeutic regimen management, Readiness for
    enhanced
Therapeutic regimen management, Ineffective community
Therapeutic regimen management, Ineffective family
Thermoregulation, Ineffective
Thought processes, Disturbed

Continued

BOX **4-2**

NANDA-Approved Nursing Diagnoses—cont'd

Tissue integrity, Impaired
Tissue perfusion, Ineffective
Transfer ability, Impaired
Trauma, Risk for
Urinary elimination, Impaired
Urinary elimination, Readiness for enhanced
Urinary retention
Ventilation, Impaired spontaneous
Ventilatory weaning response, Dysfunctional
Violence, Risk for other-directed
Violence, Risk for self-directed
Walking, Impaired
Wandering

Medical Diagnosis

A medical diagnosis is the **health problem or disease state** of the patient. In the medical model of psychiatry, health problems are the mental disorders classified in the *Diagnostic and Statistical Manual of Mental Disorders*, ed 4, text revised (DSM-IV-TR). In the DSM-IV-TR the individual is evaluated on each of the following axes (Box 4-3):

- Axis I Clinical disorders
- Axis II Personality disorders
- Axis III General medical conditions
- Axis IV Psychosocial and environmental problems
- Axis V Global assessment and functioning

BOX **4-3**

DSM-IV-TR CLASSIFICATION

NOS = Not Otherwise Specified.

An x appearing in a diagnostic code indicates that a specific code number is required.

An ellipsis (. . .) is used in the names of certain disorders to indicate that the name of a specific mental disorder or general medical condition should be inserted when recording the name (e.g., 293.0 Delirium Due to Hypothyroidism).

If criteria are currently met, one of the following severity specifiers may be noted after the diagnosis:

Mild

Moderate

Severe

If criteria are no longer met, one of the following specifiers may be noted:

In Partial Remission

In Full Remission

Prior History

Axis I Clinical Disorders

Disorders usually first diagnosed in infancy, childhood, or adolescence

Mental retardation

NOTE: These are coded on Axis II.

317	Mild Mental Retardation
318.0	Moderate Mental Retardation
318.1	Severe Mental Retardation
318.2	Profound Mental Retardation
319	Mental Retardation, Severity Unspecified

Learning disorders

315.00	Reading Disorders
315.1	Mathematics Disorder
315.2	Disorder of Written Expression
315.9	Learning Disorder NOS

Motor skills disorder

315.4	Developmental Coordination Disorder

Continued

BOX **4-3**

DSM-IV-TR CLASSIFICATION—cont'd

Communication disorders

315.31	Expressive Language Disorder
315.31	Mixed Receptive-Expressive Language Disorder
315.39	Phonological Disorder
307.0	Stuttering

Pervasive developmental disorders

307.9	Communication Disorder NOS
299.00	Autistic Disorder
299.80	Rett's Disorder
299.10	Childhood Disintegrative Disorder
299.80	Asperger's Disorder
299.80	Pervasive Developmental Disorder NOS

Attention-deficit and disruptive behavior disorders

314.xx	Attention-Deficit/Hyperactivity Disorder
.01	Combined Type
.00	Predominantly Inattentive Type
.01	Predominantly Hyperactive-Impulsive Type
314.9	Attention-Deficit/Hyperactivity Disorders NOS
312.8	Conduct Disorder
	Specify type: Childhood-Onset Type/Adolescent-Onset Type
313.81	Oppositional Defiant Disorder
312.9	Disruptive Behavior Disorder NOS

Feeding and eating disorders of infancy or early childhood

307.52	Pica
307.53	Rumination Disorder
307.59	Feeding Disorder of Infancy or Early Childhood

Tic disorders

307.23	Tourette's Disorder
307.22	Chronic Motor or Vocal Tic Disorder

From American Psychiatric Association: Diagnostic and statistical manual of mental disorders, *ed 4, text revision (DSM-IV-TR), Washington, DC, 2000, The Association.*

DSM-IV-TR CLASSIFICATION—cont'd

Tic disorders—cont'd

307.21   Transient Tic Disorder
         Specify if: Single Episode/Recurrent
307.20   Tic Disorder NOS

Elimination disorders

___._   Encopresis
787.6   With Constipation and Overflow Incontinence
307.7   Without Constipation and Overflow Incontinence
307.6   Enuresis (Not Due to a General Medical Condition)
         Specify type: Nocturnal Only/Diurnal Only/Nocturnal
         and Diurnal

Other disorders of infancy, childhood, or adolescence

309.21   Separation Anxiety Disorder
         Specify if: Early Onset
313.89   Reactive Attachment Disorder of Infancy or Early
         Childhood
         Specify type: Inhibited Type/Disinhibited Type
307.3   Stereotypic Movement Disorder
         Specify if: With Self-Injurious Behavior
313.9   Disorder of Infancy, Childhood, or Adolescence NOS

Delirium, dementia, and amnestic and other cognitive disorders

Delirium

293.0   Delirium Due to . . . *[Indicate the General Medical
         Condition]*
___._   Substance Intoxication Delirium *(refer to Substance-
         Related Disorders for substance-specific codes)*
___._   Substance Withdrawal Delirium *(refer to Substance-
         Related Disorders for substance-specific codes)*
___._   Delirium Due to Multiple Etiologies *(code each of the
         specific etiologies)*
780.09   Delirium NOS

Continued

.DSM-IV-TR CLASSIFICATION—cont'd

Dementia

290.xx	Dementia of the Alzheimer's Type, With Early Onset *(also code 331.0 Alzheimer's disease on Axis III)*
.10	Uncomplicated
.11	With Delirium
.12	With Delusions
.13	With Depressed Mood
	Specify if: With Behavioral Disturbance
290.xx	Dementia of the Alzheimer's Type, With Late Onset *(also code 331.0 Alzheimer's disease on Axis III)*
.0	Uncomplicated
.3	With Delirium
.20	With Delusions
.21	With Depressed Mood
	Specify if: With Behavioral Disturbance
290.xx	Vascular Dementia
.40	Uncomplicated
.41	With Delirium
.42	With Delusions
.43	With Depressed Mood
	Specify if: With Behavioral Disturbance
294.9	Dementia Due to HIV Disease *(also code 043.1 HIV infection affecting central nervous system on Axis III)*
294.1	Dementia Due to Head Trauma *(also code 854.00 head injury on Axis III)*
294.1	Dementia Due to Parkinson's Disease *(also code 332.0 Parkinson's disease on Axis III)*
294.1	Dementia Due to Huntington's Disease *(also code 333.4 Huntington's disease on Axis III)*
290.10	Dementia Due to Pick's Disease *(also code 331.1 Pick's disease on Axis III)*
290.10	Dementia Due to Creutzfeldt-Jakob Disease *(also code 046.1 Creutzfeldt-Jakob disease on Axis III)*

From American Psychiatric Association: Diagnostic and statistical manual of mental disorders, *ed 4, text revision (DSM-IV-TR), Washington, DC, 2000, The Association.*

DSM-IV-TR CLASSIFICATION—cont'd

Dementia—cont'd

294.1   Dementia Due to . . . *[indicate the General Medical Condition not listed above] (also code the general medical condition on Axis III)*

___.___   Substance-Induced Persisting Dementia *(refer to Substance-Related Disorders for substance-specific codes)*

___.___   Dementia Due to Multiple Etiologies *(code each of the specific etiologies)*

294.8   Dementia NOS

Amnestic disorders

294.0   Amnestic Disorder Due to . . . *[Indicate the General Medical Condition]*
Specify if: Transient/Chronic

___.___   Substance-Induced Persisting Amnestic Disorder *(refer to Substance-Related Disorders for substance-specific codes)*

294.8   Amnestic Disorder NOS

Other cognitive disorders

294.9   Cognitive Disorders NOS

Mental disorders due to a general medical condition not elsewhere classified

293.89   Catatonic Disorder Due to . . . *[Indicate the General Medical Condition]*

310.1   Personality Change Due to . . . *[Indicate the General Medical Condition]*
Specify type: Labile Type/Disinhibited Type/Aggressive Type/Apathetic Type/Paranoid Type/Other Type/Combined Type/Unspecified Type

293.9   Mental Disorder NOS Due to . . . *[Indicate the General Medical Condition]*

Continued

DSM-IV-TR CLASSIFICATION—cont'd

Substance-related disorders

[a]The following specifiers may be applied to Substance Dependence:
  With Physiological Dependence/Without Physiological
    Dependence
  Early Full Remission/Early Partial Remission
  Sustained Full Remission/Sustained Partial Remission
  On Agonist Therapy/In a Controlled Environment
*The following specifiers apply to Substance-Induced Disorders as
  noted:*
  [I]With Onset During Intoxication/[W]With Onset During Withdrawal

Alcohol-related disorders

Alcohol use disorders
  303.90   Alcohol Dependence[a]
  305.00   Alcohol Abuse

Alcohol-induced disorders
  303.00   Alcohol Intoxication
  291.8   Alcohol Withdrawal
            Specify if: With Perceptual Disturbances
  291.0   Alcohol Intoxication Delirium
  291.0   Alcohol Withdrawal Delirium
  291.2   Alcohol-Induced Persisting Dementia
  291.1   Alcohol-Induced Persisting Amnestic Disorder
  291.x   Alcohol-Induced Psychotic Disorder
    .5   With Delusions[I,W]
    .3   With Hallucinations[I,W]
  291.8   Alcohol-Induced Mood Disorder[I,W]
  291.8   Alcohol-Induced Anxiety Disorder[I,W]
  291.8   Alcohol-Induced Sexual Dysfunction[I]
  291.8   Alcohol-Induced Sleep Disorder[I,W]
  291.9   Alcohol-Related Disorder NOS

Amphetamine (or amphetamine-like)-related disorders

Amphetamine use disorders
  304.40   Amphetamine Dependence[a]
  305.70   Amphetamine Abuse

DSM-IV-TR CLASSIFICATION—cont'd

Amphetamine-induced disorders
292.89	Amphetamine Intoxication
	Specify if: With Perceptual Disturbances
292.0	Amphetamine Withdrawal
292.81	Amphetamine Intoxication Delirium
292.xx	Amphetamine-Induced Psychotic Disorders
.11	With Delusions[I]
.12	With Hallucinations[I]
292.84	Amphetamine-Induced Mood Disorder[I,W]
292.89	Amphetamine-Induced Anxiety Disorder[I]
292.89	Amphetamine-Induced Sexual Dysfunction[I]
292.89	Amphetamine-Induced Sleep Disorder[I,W]
292.9	Amphetamine-Induced Disorder NOS

Caffeine-related disorders
Caffeine-induced disorders
305.90	Caffeine Intoxication
292.89	Caffeine-Induced Anxiety Disorder[I]
292.89	Caffeine-Induced Sleep Disorder[I]
292.9	Caffeine-Related Disorder NOS

Cannabis-related disorders
Cannabis use disorders
304.30	Cannabis Dependence[a]
305.20	Cannabis Abuse

Cannabis-induced disorders
292.89	Cannabis Intoxication
	Specify if: Perceptual Disturbances
292.81	Cannabis Intoxication Delirium
292.xx	Cannabis-Induced Psychotic Disorder
.11	With Delusions[I]
.12	With Hallucinations[I]
292.89	Cannabis-Induced Anxiety Disorder[I]
292.9	Cannabis-Related Disorder NOS

Continued

DSM-IV-TR CLASSIFICATION—cont'd

Cocaine-related disorders
Cocaine use disorders
304.20   Cocaine Dependence[a]
305.60   Cocaine Abuse
Cocaine-induced disorders
292.89   Cocaine intoxication
          Specify if: With Perceptual Disturbances
292.0   Cocaine Withdrawal
292.81   Cocaine Intoxication Delirium
292.xx   Cocaine-Induced Psychotic Disorder
   .11   With Delusions[I]
   .12   With Hallucinations[I]
292.84   Cocaine-Induced Mood Disorder[I,W]
292.89   Cocaine-Induced Anxiety Disorder[I,W]
292.89   Cocaine-Induced Sexual Dysfunction[I,W]
292.89   Cocaine-Induced Sleep Disorder[I,W]
292.9   Cocaine-Related Disorder NOS

Hallucinogen-related disorders
Hallucinogen use disorders
304.50   Hallucinogen Dependence[a]
305.30   Hallucinogen Abuse
Hallucinogen-induced disorders
292.89   Hallucinogen Intoxication
292.89   Hallucinogen Persisting Perception Disorder (Flashbacks)
292.81   Hallucinogen Intoxication Delirium
292.xx   Hallucinogen-Induced Psychotic Disorder
          Hallucinogen Intoxication Delirium
   .11   With Delusions[I]
   .12   With Hallucinations[I]
292.84   Hallucinogen-Induced Mood Disorders[I]
292.89   Hallucinogen-Induced Anxiety Disorder[I]
292.9   Hallucinogen-Related Disorder NOS

DSM-IV-TR CLASSIFICATION—cont'd

Inhalant-related disorders
Inhalant use disorders
304.60   Inhalant Dependence[a]
305.90   Inhalant Abuse
292.89   Inhalant Intoxication
292.81   Inhalant Intoxication Delirium
292.82   Inhalant-Induced Persisting Dementia
292.xx   Inhalant-Induced Psychotic Disorder
.11   With Delusions[I]
.12   With Hallucinations[I]
292.84   Inhalant-Induced Mood Disorder
292.89   Inhalant-Induced Anxiety Disorder
292.9   Inhalant-Related Disorder NOS

Nicotine-related disorders
Nicotine use disorders
305.10   Nicotine Dependence[a]
Nicotine-induced disorders
292.0   Nicotine Withdrawal
292.9   Nicotine-Related Disorder NOS

Opioid-related disorders
Opioid use disorders
304.00   Opioid Dependence[a]
305.50   Opioid Abuse
Opioid-induced disorders
292.89   Opioid Intoxication
Specify if: With Perceptual Disturbances
292.0   Opioid Withdrawal
292.81   Opioid-Intoxication Delirium
292.xx   Opioid-Induced Psychotic Disorder
.11   With Delusions[I]
.12   With Hallucinations[I]
292.84   Opioid-Induced Mood Disorder[I]
292.89   Opioid-Induced Sexual Dysfunction[I,W]
292.89   Opioid-Induced Sleep Disorder[I]
292.9   Opioid-Related Disorder NOS

Continued

DSM-IV-TR CLASSIFICATION—cont'd

Phencyclidine-related (or phencyclidine-like) disorders
Phencyclidine use disorders
   304.90   Phencyclidine Dependence[a]
   305.90   Phencyclidine Abuse
Phencyclidine-induced disorders
   292.89   Phencyclidine Intoxication
             Specify if: With Perceptual Disturbances
   292.81   Phencyclidine Intoxication Delirium
   292.xx   Phencyclidine-Induced Psychotic Disorder
     .11   With Delusions[I]
     .12   With Hallucinations[I]
   292.84   Phencyclidine-Induced Mood Disorder[I]
   292.89   Phencyclidine-Induced Anxiety Disorder[I]
   292.9   Phencyclidine-Related Disorder NOS

Sedative-, hypnotic-, or anxiolytic-related disorders
Sedative, hypnotic, or anxiolytic use disorders
   304.10   Sedative, Hypnotic, or Anxiolytic Dependence[a]
   305.40   Sedative, Hypnotic, or Anxiolytic Abuse
Sedative-, hypnotic-, or anxiolytic-induced disorders
   292.89   Sedative, Hypnotic, or Anxiolytic Intoxication
   292.0   Sedative, Hypnotic, or Anxiolytic Withdrawal
             Specify if: With Perceptual Disturbances
   292.81   Sedative, Hypnotic, or Anxiolytic Intoxication Delirium
   292.81   Sedative, Hypnotic, or Anxiolytic Withdrawal Delirium
   292.82   Sedative-, Hypnotic-, or Anxiolytic-Induced Persisting Dementia
   292.83   Sedative-, Hypnotic-, or Anxiolytic-Induced Persisting Amnestic Disorder
   292.xx   Sedative-, Hypnotic-, or Anxiolytic-Induced Psychotic Disorder
     .11   With Delusions[I,W]
     .12   With Hallucinations[I,W]
   292.84   Sedative-, Hypnotic-, or Anxiolytic-Induced Mood Disorder[I,W]

From American Psychiatric Association: Diagnostic and statistical manual of mental disorders, *ed 4, text revision (DSM-IV-TR), Washington, DC, 2000, The Association.*

DSM-IV-TR CLASSIFICATION—cont'd

Sedative-, hypnotic-, or anxiolytic-related disorders—cont'd

292.89	Sedative-, Hypnotic-, or Anxiolytic-Induced Anxiety Disorder[W]
292.89	Sedative-, Hypnotic-, or Anxiolytic-Induced Sexual Dysfunction[I]
292.89	Sedative-, Hypnotic-, or Anxiolytic-Induced Sleep Disorder[I,W]
292.9	Sedative-, Hypnotic-, or Anxiolytic-Related Disorder NOS

Polysubstance-related disorder

304.80	Polysubstance Dependence[a]

Other (or unknown) substance-related disorders

Other (or unknown) substance use disorders

304.90	Other (or Unknown) Substance Dependence[a]
305.90	Other (or Unknown) Substance Abuse

Other (or unknown) substance-induced disorders

292.89	Other (or Unknown) Substance Intoxication *Specify if:* With Perceptual Disturbances
292.0	Other (or Unknown) Substance Withdrawal *Specify if:* With Perceptual Disturbances
292.81	Other (or Unknown) Substance-Induced Delirium
292.82	Other (or Unknown) Substance-Induced Persisting Dementia
292.83	Other (or Unknown) Substance-Induced Persisting Amnestic Disorder
292.xx	Other (or Unknown) Substance-Induced Psychotic Disorder
.11	With Delusions[I,W]
.12	With Hallucinations[I,W]
292.84	Other (or Unknown) Substance-Induced Mood Disorder[I,W]
292.89	Other (or Unknown) Substance-Induced Anxiety Disorder[I,W]
292.89	Other (or Unknown) Substance-Induced Anxiety Sexual Dysfunction[I]

Continued

DSM-IV-TR CLASSIFICATION—cont'd

Other (or unknown) substance-related disorders—cont'd

292.89   Other (or Unknown) Substance-Induced Sleep Disorder[I,W]

292.9   Other (or Unknown) Substance-Related Disorder NOS

Schizophrenia and other psychotic disorders

295.xx   Schizophrenia

The following Classification of Longitudinal Course applies to all subtypes of Schizophrenia:

     Episodic With Interepisode Residual Symptoms (*specify if:* With Prominent Negative Symptoms)/Episodic With No Interepisode Residual Symptoms/Continuous (*specify if:* With Prominent Negative Symptoms)

     Single Episode in Partial Remission (*specify if:* With Prominent Negative Symptoms/Single Episode in Full Remission)

     Other or Unspecified Pattern

     .30   Paranoid Type

     .10   Disorganized Type

     .20   Catatonic Type

     .90   Undifferentiated Type

     .60   Residual Type

295.40   Schizophreniform Disorder

     Specify if: Without Good Prognostic Features/With Good Prognostic Features

295.70   Schizoaffective Disorder

     Specify type: Bipolar Type/Depressive Type

297.1   Delusional Disorder

     Specify type: Erotomanic Type/Grandiose Type/Jealous Type/Persecutory Type/Somatic Type/Mixed Type/Unspecified Type

298.8   Brief Psychotic Disorder

     Specify if: With Marked Stressor(s)/Without Marked Stressor(s)/With Postpartum Onset

297.3   Shared Psychotic Disorder

From American Psychiatric Association: Diagnostic and statistical manual of mental disorders, *ed 4, text revision (DSM-IV-TR), Washington, DC, 2000, The Association.*

DSM-IV-TR CLASSIFICATION—cont'd

Schizophrenia and other psychotic disorders—cont'd

293.xx	Psychotic Disorder Due to . . . [Indicate the General Medical Condition]
.81	With Delusions
.82	With Hallucinations
___._	Substance-Induced Psychotic Disorder (refer to Substance-Related Disorders for substance-specific codes)
	Specify if: With Onset During Intoxication/With Onset During Withdrawal
298.9	Psychotic Disorder NOS

Mood disorders

Code current state of Major Depressive Disorder or Bipolar I Disorder in fifth digit:

1 = Mild
2 = Moderate
3 = Severe, Without Psychotic Features
4 = Severe, With Psychotic Features
    Specify: Mood-Congruent Psychotic Features/Mood-Incongruent Psychotic Features
5 = In Partial Remission
6 = In Full Remission
0 = Unspecified

The following specifiers apply (for current or most recent episode) to Mood Disorders as noted:
[a]Severity/Psychotic/Remission Specifiers/[b]Chronic/[c]With Catatonic Features/[d]With Melancholic Features/[e]With Atypical Features/[f]With Postpartum Onset

The following specifiers apply to Mood Disorders as noted:
[g]With or Without Full Interepisode Recovery/
[h]With Seasonal Pattern/[i]With Rapid Cycling

Depressive disorders

296.xx	Major Depressive Disorder
.2x	Single Episode[a,b,c,d,e,f]
.3x	Recurrent[a,b,c,d,e,f,g,h]

Continued

DSM-IV-TR CLASSIFICATION—cont'd

300.4	Dysthymic Disorder
	Specify if: Early Onset/Late Onset
	Specify if: With Atypical Features
311	Depressive Disorder NOS

Bipolar disorders

296.xx	Bipolar I Disorder.
.0x	Single Manic Episode[a,c,f]
	Specify if: Mixed
.40	Most Recent Episode Hypomanic[g,h,i]
.4x	Most Recent Episode Manic[a,c,f,g,h,i]
.6x	Most Recent Episode Mixed[a,c,f,g,h,i]
.5x	Most Recent Episode Depressed[a,b,c,d,e,f,g,h,i]
.7	Most Recent Episode Unspecified[g,h,i]
296.89	Bipolar II Disorder[a,b,c,d,e,f,g,h,i]
	Specify (current or most recent episode): Hypomanic/Depressed
301.13	Cyclothymic Disorder
296.80	Bipolar Disorder NOS
293.83	Mood Disorder Due to . . . *[Indicate the General Medical Condition]*
	Specify type: With Depressive Features/With Major Depressive-Like Episode/With Manic Features/With Mixed Features
__.__	Substance-Induced Mood Disorder *[refer to Substance-Related Disorders for substance-specific codes]*
	Specify type: With Depressive Features/With Manic Features/With Mixed Features
	Specify if: With Onset During Intoxication/With Onset During Withdrawal
296.90	Mood Disorder NOS

Anxiety disorders

300.01	Panic Disorder Without Agoraphobia
300.21	Panic Disorder With Agoraphobia

From American Psychiatric Association: Diagnostic and statistical manual of mental disorders, *ed 4, text revision (DSM-IV-TR), Washington, DC, 2000, The Association.*

DSM-IV-TR CLASSIFICATION—cont'd

Anxiety disorders—cont'd

300.22	Agoraphobia Without History of Panic Disorder
300.29	Specific Phobia
	Specify type: Animal Type/Natural Environment Type/ Blood-Injection-Injury Type/Situational Type/Other Type
300.23	Social Phobia
	Specify if: Generalized
300.3	Obsessive-Compulsive Disorder
	Specify if: With Poor Insight
309.81	Posttraumatic Stress Disorder
	Specify if: Acute/Chronic
	Specify if: With Delayed Onset
308.3	Acute Stress Disorder
300.02	Generalized Anxiety Disorder
293.89	Anxiety Disorder Due to . . . *[Indicate the General Medical Condition]*
	Specify if: With Generalized Anxiety/With Panic Attacks/ With Obsessive-Compulsive Symptoms
__.__	Substance-Induced Anxiety Disorder *[refer to Substance-Related Disorders for substance-specific codes]*
	Specify if: With Generalized Anxiety/With Panic Attacks/ With Obsessive-Compulsive Symptoms/With Phobic Symptoms
	Specify if: With Onset During Intoxication/With Onset During Withdrawal
300.00	Anxiety Disorder NOS

Somatoform disorders

300.81	Somatization Disorder
300.81	Undifferentiated Somatoform Disorder
300.11	Conversion Disorder
	Specify if: With Motor Symptom or Deficit/With Sensory Symptom or Deficit/With Seizures or Convulsions/With Mixed Presentation
307.xx	Pain Disorder
.80	Associated With Psychological Factors

Continued

DSM-IV-TR CLASSIFICATION—cont'd

Anxiety disorders—cont'd

.89	Associated With Both Psychological Factors and a General Medical Condition
	Specify if: Acute/Chronic
300.7	Hypochondriasis
	Specify if: With Poor Insight
300.7	Body Dysmorphic Disorder
300.89	Somatoform Disorder NOS

Factitious disorders

300.xx	Factitious Disorder
.16	With Predominantly Psychological Signs and Symptoms
.19	With Predominantly Physical Signs and Symptoms
.19	With Combined Psychological and Physical Signs and Symptoms
300.19	Factitious Disorder NOS

Dissociative disorders

300.12	Dissociative Amnesia
300.13	Dissociative Fugue
300.14	Dissociative Identity Disorder
300.6	Depersonalization Disorder
300.15	Dissociative Disorder NOS

Sexual and gender identity disorders

Sexual dysfunctions

The following specifiers apply to all primary Sexual Dysfunctions:
Lifelong Type/Acquired Type/Generalized Type/Situational Type
Due to Psychological Factors/Due to Combined Factors

Sexual desire disorders

302.71	Hypoactive Sexual Desire Disorder
302.79	Sexual Aversion Disorder

From American Psychiatric Association: Diagnostic and statistical manual of mental disorders, *ed 4, text revision (DSM-IV-TR), Washington, DC, 2000, The Association.*

DSM-IV-TR CLASSIFICATION—cont'd

Sexual arousal disorders

302.72   Female Sexual Arousal Disorder
302.72   Male Erectile Disorder

Orgasm disorders

302.73   Female Orgasmic Disorder
302.74   Male Orgasmic Disorder
302.75   Premature Ejaculation

Sexual pain disorders

302.76   Dyspareunia (Not Due to a General Medical Condition)
306.51   Vaginismus (Not Due to a General Medical Condition)

Sexual dysfunctions due to a general medical condition

625.8   Female Hypoactive Sexual Desire Disorder Due to . . .
         [Indicate the General Medical Condition]
609.89   Male Hypoactive Sexual Desire Disorder Due to . . .
         [Indicate the General Medical Condition]
607.84   Male Erectile Disorder Due to . . . *[Indicate the General
         Medical Condition]*
625.0   Female Dyspareunia Due to . . . *[Indicate the General
         Medical Condition]*
608.89   Male Dyspareunia Due to . . . *[Indicate the General
         Medical Condition]*
625.8   Other Female Sexual Dysfunction Due to . . . *[Indicate
         the General Medical Condition]*
608.89   Other Male Sexual Dysfunction Due to . . . *[Indicate the
         General Medical Condition]*
___.___ Substance-Induced Sexual Dysfunction (refer to
         Substance-Related Disorders for substance-specific
         codes)
         Specify if: With Impaired Desired/With Impaired
         Arousal/With Impaired Orgasm/With Sexual Pain
         Specify if: With Onset During Intoxication
302.70   Sexual Dysfunction NOS

Paraphilias

302.4   Exhibitionism
302.81   Fetishism

Continued

DSM-IV-TR CLASSIFICATION—cont'd

Paraphilias—cont'd

302.89	Frotteurism
302.2	Pedophilia

Specify if: Sexually Attracted to Males/Sexually Attracted to Females/Sexually Attracted to Both
Specify type: Exclusive Type/Nonexclusive Type

302.83	Sexual Masochism
302.84	Sexual Sadism
302.3	Transvestic Fetishism

Specify if: With Gender Dysphoria

302.82	Voyeurism
302.9	Paraphilia NOS

Gender identity disorders

3022.xx	Gender Identity Disorder
.6	In Children
.85	In Adolescents or Adults

Specify if: Sexually Attracted to Males/Sexually Attracted to Females/Sexually Attracted to Both/Sexually Attracted to Neither

302.6	Gender Identity Disorder NOS
302.9	Sexual Disorder NOS

Eating disorders

307.1	Anorexia nervosa

Specify type: Restricting Type: Binge-Eating/Purging Type

307.51	Bulimia Nervosa

Specify type: Purging Type/Nonpurging Type

307.50	Eating Disorder NOS

Sleep Disorders

Primary sleep disorders

Dyssomnias

307.42	Primary Insomnia

From American Psychiatric Association: Diagnostic and statistical manual of mental disorders, ed 4, text revision (DSM-IV-TR), Washington, DC, 2000, The Association.

DSM-IV-TR CLASSIFICATION—cont'd

Primary sleep disorders—cont'd

307.44	Primary Hypersomnia
	Specify if: Recurrent
347	Narcolepsy
780.59	Breathing-Related Sleep Disorder
307.45	Circadian Rhythm Sleep Disorder
	Specify type: Delayed Sleep Phase Type/Jet Lag Type/ Shift Work Type/Unspecified Type
307.47	Dyssomnias NOS

Parasomnias

307.47	Nightmare Disorder
307.46	Sleep Terror Disorder
307.46	Sleepwalking Disorder
307.47	Parasomnia NOS

Sleep disorders related to another mental disorder

307.42	Insomnia Related to . . . *[Indicate the Axis I or Axis II Disorder]*
307.44	Hypersomnia Related to . . . *[Indicate the Axis I or Axis II Disorder]*

Other sleep disorders

780.xx	Sleep Disorder Due to . . . *[Indicate the General Medical Condition]*
.52	Insomnia Type
.54	Hypersomnia Type
.59	Parasomnia Type
.59	Mixed Type
___.__	Substance-Induced Sleep Disorder (refer to Substance-Related Disorders for substance-specific codes) *Specify type:* Insomnia Type/Hypersomnia Type/ Parasomnia Type/Mixed Type *Specify if:* With Onset During Intoxication/With Onset During Withdrawal

Impulse control disorders not elsewhere classified

312.34	Intermittent Explosive Disorder

Continued

DSM-IV-TR CLASSIFICATION—cont'd

Impulse control disorders not elsewhere classified—cont'd

312.32	Kleptomania
312.33	Pyromania
312.31	Pathological Gambling
312.39	Trichotillomania
312.3	Impulse Control Disorder NOS

Adjustment disorders

309.xx	Adjustment Disorder
.0	With Depressed Mood
.24	With Anxiety
.28	With Mixed Anxiety and Depressed Mood
.3	With Disturbance of Conduct
.4	With Mixed Disturbance of Emotions and Conduct
.9	Unspecified
	Specify if: Acute/Chronic

Personality disorders

NOTE: These are coded on Axis II.

301.0	Paranoid Personality Disorder
301.20	Schizoid Personality Disorder
301.22	Schizotypal Personality Disorder
301.7	Antisocial Personality Disorder
301.83	Borderline Personality Disorder
301.50	Histrionic Personality Disorder
301.81	Narcissistic Personality Disorder
301.82	Avoidant Personality Disorder
301.6	Dependent Personality Disorder
301.4	Obsessive-Compulsive Personality Disorder
301.9	Personality Disorder NOS

Other conditions that may be a focus of clinical attention

Psychological factors affecting medical condition

. . . *[Specified Psychological Factor]* . . . affecting *[Indicate the General Medical Condition]* Choose name based on nature of factors:

From American Psychiatric Association: Diagnostic and statistical manual of mental disorders, *ed 4, text revision (DSM-IV-TR), Washington, DC, 2000, The Association.*

DSM-IV-TR CLASSIFICATION—cont'd

Psychological factors affecting medical condition—cont'd

Mental Disorder Affecting Medical Condition
Psychological Symptoms Affecting Medical Condition
Personality Traits or Coping Style Affecting Medical Condition
Maladaptive Health Behaviors Affecting Medical Condition
Stress-Related Physiological Response Affecting Medical Condition
Other or Unspecified Psychological Factors Affecting Medical
   Condition

Medication-induced movement disorders

332.1	Neuroleptic-Induced Parkinsonism
333.92	Neuroleptic Malignant Syndrome
333.7	Neuroleptic-Induced Acute Dystonia
333.99	Neuroleptic-Induced Acute Akathisia
333.82	Neuroleptic-Induced Tardive Dyskinesia
333.1	Medication-Induced Postural Tremor
333.90	Medication-Induced Movement Disorder NOS

Other medication-induced disorders

995.2	Adverse Effects of Medication NOS

Relational problems

V61.9	Relational Problem Related to a Mental Disorder or General Medical Condition
V61.20	Parent-Child Relational Problem
V61.1	Partner Relational Problem
V61.8	Sibling Relational Problem
V62.81	Relational Problem NOS

Problems related to abuse or neglect

V61.21	Physical Abuse of Child (code 995.5 if focus of attention is on victim)
V61.21	Sexual Abuse of Child (code 995.5 if focus of attention is on victim)
V61.21	Neglect of Child (code 995.5 if focus of attention is on victim)
V61.1	Physical Abuse of Adult (code 995.81 if focus of attention is on victim)

Continued

DSM-IV-TR CLASSIFICATION—cont'd

Problems related to abuse or neglect—cont'd

V61.1	Sexual Abuse of Adult (code 995.81 if focus of attention is on victim)

Additional conditions that may be a focus of clinical attention

V15.81	Noncompliance With Treatment
V65.2	Malingering
V71.01	Adult Antisocial Behavior
V71.02	Childhood or Adolescent Antisocial Behavior
V62.89	Borderline Intellectual Functioning
	NOTE: This is coded on Axis II.
780.9	Age-Related Cognitive Decline
V62.82	Bereavement
V62.3	Academic Problem
V62.2	Occupational Problem
313.82	Identity Problem
V62.89	Religious or Spiritual Problem
V62.4	Acculturation Problem
V62.89	Phase of Life Problem

Additional codes

300.9	Unspecified Mental Disorder (nonpsychotic)
V71.09	No Diagnosis or Condition on Axis I
799.9	Diagnosis or Condition Deferred on Axis I
V71.09	No Diagnosis on Axis II
799.9	Diagnosis Deferred on Axis II

Axis II Personality Disorders

301.0	Paranoid Personality Disorder
301.20	Schizoid Personality Disorder
301.22	Schizotypal Personality Disorder
301.7	Antisocial Personality Disorder
301.83	Borderline Personality Disorder
301.5	Histrionic Personality Disorder
301.81	Narcissistic Personality Disorder
301.82	Avoidant Personality Disorder

From American Psychiatric Association: Diagnostic and statistical manual of mental disorders, *ed 4, text revision (DSM-IV-TR), Washington, DC, 2000, The Association.*

DSM-IV-TR CLASSIFICATION—cont'd

Axis II Personality Disorders—cont'd

301.65	Dependent Personality Disorder
301.45	Obsessive-Compulsive Personality Disorder
301.9	Personality Disorder NOS

Axis III General Medical Conditions (with ICD-9-CM codes)

Infectious and Parasitic Diseases (001-139)

Neoplasms (140-239)

Endocrine, Nutritional, and Metabolic Diseases and Immunity Disorders (240-279)

Diseases of the Blood and Blood-Forming Organs (280-289)

Diseases of the Nervous System and Sense Organs (320-389)

Diseases of the Circulatory System (390-459)

Diseases of the Respiratory System (460-519)

Diseases of the Digestive System (520-579)

Diseases of the Genitourinary System (580-629)

Complications of Pregnancy, Childbirth, and the Puerperium (630-676)

Diseases of the Skin and Subcutaneous Tissue (680-709)

Diseases of the Musculoskeletal System and Connective Tissue (710-739)

Congenital Anomalies (740-759)

Certain Conditions Originating in the Perinatal Period (760-779)

Symptoms, Signs, and Ill-Defined Conditions (780-799)

Injury and Poisoning (800-999)

Axis IV Psychosocial and Environmental Problems

- **Problems with primary support group**—e.g., death of a family member; health problems in family; disruption of family by separation, divorce, or estrangement; removal from the home; remarriage of parent; sexual or physical abuse; parental overprotection; neglect of child; inadequate discipline; discord with siblings; birth of a sibling
- **Problems related to the social environment**—e.g., death or loss of friend; inadequate social support; living alone; difficulty with acculturation; discrimination; adjustment to life cycle transition (e.g., retirement)

Continued

DSM-IV-TR CLASSIFICATION—cont'd

Axis IV Psychosocial and Environmental Problems—cont'd

- **Educational problems**—e.g., illiteracy; academic problems; discord with teachers or classmates; inadequate school environment
- **Occupational problems**—e.g., unemployment; threat of job loss; stressful work schedule; difficult work conditions; job dissatisfaction; job change; discord with boss or co-workers
- **Housing problems**—e.g., homelessness; inadequate housing; unsafe neighborhood; discord with neighbors or landlord
- **Economic problems**—e.g., extreme poverty; inadequate finances; insufficient welfare support
- **Problems with access to health care services**—e.g., inadequate health care services; transportation to health care facilities unavailable; inadequate health insurance
- **Problems related to interaction with the legal system crime**—e.g., arrest; incarceration; litigation; victim of crime

Axis V Global Assessment of Functioning (GAF) Scale*

Consider psychological, social, and occupational functioning on a hypothetical continuum of mental health-illness. Do not include impairment in functioning due to physical (or environmental) limitations.

Code (NOTE: Use intermediate codes when appropriate, e.g., 45, 68, 72.)

100	Superior functioning in a wide range of activities, life's
|	problems never seem to get out of hand, is sought out by
91	others because of many positive qualities. No symptoms.

From American Psychiatric Association: Diagnostic and statistical manual of mental disorders, *ed 4, text revision (DSM-IV-TR), Washington, DC, 2000, The Association.*
*The rating of overall psychological functioning on a scale of 0-100 was operationalized by Luborsky in the Health-Sickness Rating Scale (Luborsky L: Arch Gen Psychiatry 7:407-417, 1962). Spitzer and colleagues developed a revision of the Health-Sickness Rating Scale called the Global Assessment Scale (GAS) (Endicott J, Spitzer RL, Fleiss JL, Cohen J: Arch Gen Psychiatry 33:766-771, 1976). A modified version of the GAS was included in DSM-III-R as the Global Assessment of Functioning (GAF) Scale.

DSM-IV-TR CLASSIFICATION—cont'd

Code

90 | 81	Absent or minimal symptoms (e.g., mild anxiety before an exam), good functioning in all areas, interested and involved in a wide range of activities, socially effective, generally satisfied with life, no more than everyday problems or concerns (e.g., an occasional argument with family members).
80 | 71	If symptoms are present, they are transient and expectable reactions to psychosocial stressors (e.g., difficulty concentrating after family argument); no more than slight impairment in social, occupational, or school functioning (e.g., temporarily falling behind in schoolwork).
70 | 61	Some mild symptoms (e.g., depressed mood and mild insomnia) OR some difficulty in social, occupational, or school functioning (e.g., occasional truancy, theft within the household), but generally functioning pretty well, has some meaningful interpersonal relationships.
60 | 51	Moderate symptoms (e.g., flat affect and circumstantial speech, occasional panic attacks) OR moderate difficulty in social, occupational, or school functioning (e.g., few friends, conflicts with peers or co-workers).
50 | 41	Serious symptoms (e.g., suicidal ideation, severe obsessional rituals, frequent shoplifting) OR any serious impairment in social, occupational, or school functioning (e.g., no friends, unable to keep a job).
40 | 31	Some impairment in reality testing or communication (e.g., speech is at times illogical, obscure, or irrelevant) OR major impairment in several areas, such as work or school, family relations, judgment, thinking, or mood (e.g., depressed man avoids friends, neglects family, and is unable to work; child frequently beats up younger children, is defiant at home, and is failing at school).

Continued

DSM-IV-TR CLASSIFICATION—cont'd

Code

30 | 21	Behavior is considerably influenced by delusions or hallucinations OR serious impairment in communication or judgment (e.g., sometimes incoherent, acts grossly inappropriately, suicidal preoccupation) OR inability to function in almost all areas (e.g., stays in bed all day; no job, home, or friends).
20 | 11	Some danger of hurting self or others (e.g., suicide attempts without clear expectation of death, frequently violent, manic excitement) OR occasionally fails to maintain minimal personal hygiene (e.g., smears feces) OR gross impairment in communication (e.g., largely incoherent or mute).
10 | 1	Persistent danger of severely hurting self or others (e.g., recurrent violence) OR persistent inability to maintain minimal personal hygiene OR serious suicidal act with clear expectation of death.
0	Inadequate information.

From American Psychiatric Association: Diagnostic and statistical manual of mental disorders, *ed 4, text revision (DSM-IV-TR), Washington, DC, 2000, The Association.*

Your Internet Connection

American Psychiatric Association
www.psych.org

Center for Mental Health Services
www.mentalhealth.org/cmhs

Internet Mental Health
www.mentalhealth.com

Mental Health Infosource
www.mhsource.com

Mental Health Net
www.mentalhelp.net

National Institute of Mental Health
www.nimh.nih.gov

Psych Central
www.psychcentral.com

U.S. Department of Health and Human Services
www.hhs.gov

Virtual Office of the Surgeon General
www.surgeongeneral.gov

▮ PRIMARY PREVENTION

Primary prevention is biological, social, or psychological intervention that promotes health and well-being or reduces the **incidence** of illness in a community by altering the causative factors before they can do harm.

Assessment of Preventive Nursing Needs

Assessment of the need for preventive nursing measures includes identification of the following:

1. **Risk factors** that if present for a person make it more likely that he or she will develop a disorder.
2. **Protective factors** that improve a person's response to stress.
3. **A target population** of individuals who are vulnerable to developing mental disorders or who may display maladaptive coping responses to specific stressors or risk factors.

Planning and Implementation

A national initiative called Healthy People 2010 has been undertaken to promote health and prevent disease in the United States. Specific nursing interventions in primary prevention include health education, environmental change, support of social systems, and stigma reduction. The overall nursing goal is to **promote constructive coping mechanisms and adaptive coping responses.**

Health Education

Health education involves strengthening individuals and groups through **building competence.** The assumption is that many maladaptive responses result from a lack of competence. This involves a lack of perceived control over one's life, a low sense of self-efficacy, a lack of effective coping strategies, and the resulting lowered self-esteem. Health education involves the following four levels of intervention:

1. Increasing the individual's or group's awareness of issues and events related to health and illness, such as normal developmental tasks
2. Increasing one's understanding of the dimensions of potential stressors, possible outcomes (both adaptive and maladaptive), and alternative coping responses
3. Increasing one's knowledge of where and how to acquire the needed resources
4. Increasing the individual's or group's problem-solving skills, interpersonal skills, tolerance of stress and frustration, motivation, hope, and self-esteem

Environmental Change

Preventive interventions may be made to modify the individual's or group's immediate environment or the larger social system. These interventions are particularly helpful when the environment has placed new demands on the patient, does not respond to developmental needs, and provides little positive reinforcement. Environmental changes may include the following types:

1. **Economic**—allocating resources for financial aid or assistance in budgeting and managing income
2. **Work**—receiving vocational testing, guidance, education, or retraining that can result in new jobs or careers
3. **Housing**—moving to new quarters, which may mean leaving or returning to family and friends; improving existing housing; gaining or losing family, friends, or roommates

   4. **Family**—attending child care facilities, nursery
      school, grade school, or camp; obtaining access to
      recreational, social, religious, or community services
   5. **Political**—influencing health care structures and
      procedures; participating in community planning and
      development; addressing legislative issues

Support of Social Systems

Strengthening social supports is a way of buffering or
cushioning the effects of a potentially stressful event. The
following four types of preventive intervention are possible:
   1. Assess communities and neighborhoods to identify
      problem areas and high-risk groups.
   2. Improve linkages between community support systems
      and formal mental health services.
   3. Strengthen existing caregiving networks, including
      church groups, civic organizations, women's groups,
      work and neighborhood supports, and self-help
      groups.
   4. Help the individual or group develop, maintain,
      expand, and use the existing social network.

Stigma Reduction

An important part of mental health promotion involves
activities related to dispelling myths and stereotypes associated with vulnerable groups, providing knowledge of normal parameters, increasing sensitivity to psychosocial factors
affecting health and illness, and enhancing the ability to give
sensitive, supportive, and humanistic health care.

   Stigma is "a cluster of negative attitudes and beliefs that
motivate the general public to fear, reject, avoid, and dis-
criminate against people with mental illness" (New Freedom
Commission on Mental Health, 2003). Unfortunately cultural stigma against mental illness is prevalent in contemporary society.

The impact of this stigma is enormous.

- Nearly two thirds of people with diagnosable mental disorders do not seek treatment, and stigma about mental illness is one of the major barriers discouraging people from seeking needed care.
- Another sign of stigma is evident in the public's reluctance to pay for mental health services and to provide the same coverage for physical and mental health care.
- Patients and their families often report that the diagnosis of a mental illness is followed by increasing isolation and loneliness as family and friends withdraw. Patients feel rejected and feared by others, and their families are met with blame.

Reducing stigma can involve the following:

- Programs of public advocacy
- Public education on mental health issues
- Contact with persons with mental illness through schools and other social institutions
- Finding causes and effective treatments for mental disorders
- Realizing that everyone encounters stress; that all people are subject to maladaptive coping responses; and that mental disorders are not the result of moral failings or limited will power, but rather they are legitimate medical illnesses that respond to specific treatments

Evaluation

The nurse should consider the following points in evaluating primary prevention interventions or programs:

1. *Efficacy.* Does the program or intervention do more good than harm in the opinion of its proponents?
2. *Effectiveness.* Does the intervention do more good than harm to its target population?

3. *Efficiency.* Is the intervention being made available to those who could benefit from it? Is there optimal use of resources?

4. *Length and timing.* Does any evidence indicate the optimal length or timing of the intervention program?

5. *Harmful effects.* Are there data to suggest that the intervention may have harmful effects (e.g., unfavorable consequences of labeling)?

6. *Screening programs.* Is there any information about the program's sensitivity, specificity, and predictive accuracy?

7. *Possible high-risk groups.* Does any evidence suggest that the program would be more efficient if it applied to a specific population at increased risk?

8. *Economic analysis.* What are the results of the cost-benefit and cost-effectiveness analyses?

◁ **Your Internet Connection**

American Public Health Association
www.apha.org

Healthy People 2010
www.healthypeople.gov

Help! Consumer's Guide to Mental Health Information
www.iComm.ca/madmagic/help/help.html

National Mental Health Association
www.nmha.org

CRISIS INTERVENTION

A crisis is an internal disturbance that results from a stressful event or a perceived threat to the self. A person's usual repertoire of coping mechanisms becomes ineffective in dealing with the threat, and the person experiences a state of disequilibrium and a rise in anxiety. The threat, or precipitating event, can usually be identified.

The goal of crisis intervention is for the person to return to the precrisis level of functioning. Crises are self-limited in time, and the intense conflict they represent can be a period of increased vulnerability, which can stimulate personal growth. What the person does with the crisis determines whether growth or disorganization results.

■ BALANCING FACTORS

In describing the resolution of a crisis, some important balancing factors need to be considered (Figure 6-1).

Successful resolution of the crisis is more likely if the individual's perception of the event is realistic rather than distorted, if situational supports are available so that others can help solve the problem, and if coping mechanisms are available to help alleviate anxiety.

■ TYPES OF CRISES

1. **Maturational crises**. These are transitional or developmental periods in a person's life during which

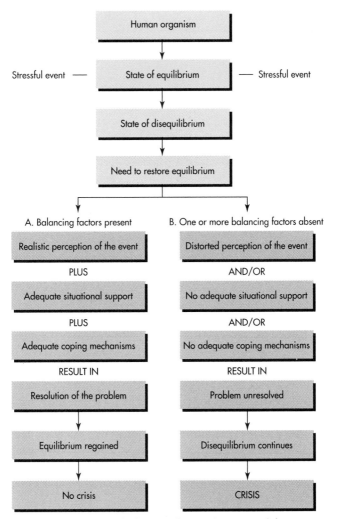

Figure 6-1 Effect of balancing factors in a stressful event. *(From Aguilera DC: Crisis intervention: theory and methodology, ed 8, St Louis, 1998, Mosby.)*

psychological equilibrium is upset, such as during
adolescence, parenthood, marriage, or retirement.
Maturational crises require role changes. The nature
and extent of the maturational crises can be
influenced by the adequacy of role models,
interpersonal resources, and the ease of others in
accepting the new role.
2. **Situational crises.** These occur when a specific
external event upsets an individual's psychological
equilibrium or a group's equilibrium. Examples
include the loss of a job, divorce, death, school
problems, illness, and disasters.

Table 6-1 presents the six phases of human disaster response.

Table 6-1	Phases of Disaster Response
PHASE	RESPONSE
Warning or threat phase	Disasters vary in the amount of warning communities receive before they occur. When no warning is given, survivors may feel more vulnerable, unsafe, and fearful of future unpredicted tragedies.
Impact phase	The greater the scope, community destruction, and personal losses associated with the disaster, the greater the psychosocial effects.
Rescue or heroic phase	In the immediate aftermath, survival, rescuing others, and promoting safety are priorities. For some, postimpact disorientation gives way to adrenaline-induced rescue behavior to save lives and protect property. Although activity level may be high, actual productivity is often low. Altruism is prominent among both survivors and emergency responders.

Continued

Table 6-1	Phases of Disaster Response—cont'd
PHASE	**RESPONSE**
Remedy or honeymoon phase	During the week to months following a disaster, formal governmental and volunteer assistance may be readily available. Community bonding occurs. Survivors may experience a short-lived sense of optimism that the help they will receive will make them whole again.
Inventory phase	Over time, survivors begin to recognize the limits of available disaster assistance. They become discouraged and physically exhausted due to enormous multiple demands, financial pressures, and the stress of relocation or living in a damaged home.
Reconstruction or recovery phase	The reconstruction of physical property and recovery of emotional well-being may continue for years following the disaster. Survivors need to readjust to and integrate new surroundings as they continue to grieve losses. Emotional resources within the family may be exhausted and social support from friends and family may be worn thin. When people come to see meaning, personal growth, and opportunity from their disaster experience, despite their losses and pain, they are well on the road to recovery. Although disasters may cause profound life-changing losses, they also bring the opportunity to recognize personal strengths and to reexamine life priorities.

ASSESSMENT

During the assessment phase the nurse must obtain data regarding the nature of the crisis and its effect. The nurse should make the following specific assessments:

1. *Identify the precipitating event,* including the needs that are threatened by the event and the point at which symptoms appeared.

2. *Identify the person's perception of the event,* including the underlying themes and memories associated with the event.

3. *Identify the nature and strength of the person's support system and coping resources,* including family, friends, and significant others who might be of help.

4. *Identify the person's previous strengths and coping mechanisms,* including successful and unsuccessful coping strategies.

PLANNING AND IMPLEMENTATION

Dynamics underlying the crisis are formulated, alternative solutions to the problem are explored, and steps for achieving the solutions are designated. This process is described in the **Patient Education Plan for coping with crisis** on page 104. *The expected outcome of nursing care is that the patient will recover from the crisis event and return to a precrisis level of functioning.* A more ambitious expected outcome would be for the patient to recover from the crisis event and attain a higher than precrisis level of functioning with improved quality of life. Four levels of crisis intervention exist, representing a hierarchy from the most basic level (level 1) to the most in-depth level (level 4):

1. *Environmental manipulation.* These interventions directly change the person's physical or interpersonal

situation for the purpose of providing situational
support or removing stress.

2. *General support.* This provides individuals with the
   feeling that the nurse is on their side and will help
   them. The nurse's demonstration of warmth,
   acceptance, empathy, and caring results in this type of
   support.

3. *Generic approach.* This type of crisis intervention is
   designed to reach individuals at high risk and large
   numbers of people as soon as possible. It applies a
   specific method to all people facing a similar crisis,
   such as assisting disaster victims to work through the
   grieving process.

4. *Individual approach.* This approach involves the
   diagnosis and treatment of a specific problem in a

 ## PATIENT EDUCATION PLAN

COPING WITH CRISIS

Content	Instructional Activities	Evaluation
Describe the crisis event	Ask about the details of the crisis, including: A timeline of the crisis Who was affected The events of the crisis Any precipitating events	Patient describes the crisis event in detail
Explore feelings, thoughts, and behaviors related to the crisis event	Determine precrisis level of functioning Discuss patient's perception of the crisis event Determine acute and long-term needs, threats, and challenges	Patient discusses precrisis level of functioning and perceptions of the crisis event Patient's needs are identified

PATIENT EDUCATION PLAN—CONT'D

COPING WITH CRISIS

Content	Instructional Activities	Evaluation
Identify coping mechanisms	Ask how stressful events have been handled in the past Analyze whether these are adaptive or maladaptive for the current crisis event Suggest additional coping strategies	Patient identifies adaptive coping mechanisms for the current crisis event
Develop a plan for coping adaptively with the crisis event	Reinforce adaptive coping mechanisms and healthy defenses With the patient, construct a coping plan for the aftermath of the crisis event	Patient develops a plan for coping with the crisis event
Assign the patient activities from coping plan	Review implementation of the coping plan Help patient generalize coping strategies for use in future crisis events	Patient reports satisfaction with coping abilities and level of functioning

specific patient. The individual approach is effective with all types of crises and in a combination of crises or when homicidal or suicidal risk exists.

The techniques of crisis intervention are active, focal, and explorative. They are not interpretive because the goal is quick resolution of an immediate problem. Table 6-2 summarizes crisis intervention techniques. Table 6-3 describes interventions for working with individuals and families with stress resulting from crises.

Table 6-2	Techniques of Crisis Intervention	
TECHNIQUE	**DEFINITION**	**EXAMPLE**
Catharsis	The release of feelings that takes place as the patient talks about emotionally charged areas	"Tell me about how you have been feeling since you lost your job."
Clarification	Encouraging the patient to express more clearly the relationship between certain events	"I've noticed that after you have an argument with your husband you become sick and can't leave your bed."
Suggestion	Influencing a person to accept an idea or belief, particularly the belief that the nurse can help and that the person will, in time, feel better	"Many other people have found it helpful to talk about this and I think you will, too."
Reinforcement of behavior	Giving the patient positive responses to adaptive behavior	"That's the first time you were able to defend yourself with your boss and it went very well. I'm so pleased that you were able to do it."
Support of defenses	Encouraging the use of healthy, adaptive defenses and discouraging those that are unhealthy or maladaptive	"Going for a bicycle ride when you were so angry was very helpful because when you returned you and your wife were able to talk things through."

Table 6-2	Techniques of Crisis Intervention—cont'd	
TECHNIQUE	**DEFINITION**	**EXAMPLE**
Raising self-esteem	Helping the patient regain feelings of self-worth	"You are a very strong person to be able to manage the family all this time. I think you will be able to handle this situation, too."
Exploration of solutions	Examining alternative ways of solving the immediate problem	"You seem to know many people in the computer field. Could you contact some of them to see whether they might know of available jobs?"

Table 6-3	Nursing Interventions for Crisis Events
TARGET AREAS	**NURSING INTERVENTIONS**
Basic Needs	Provide liaison to social agencies
Physical Deficits	Attend to physical emergencies Refer to other health care providers as necessary
Psychological Effects	
Shock	Attentively listen to telling of the crisis details
Confusion	Give nurturing support; permit regression
Denial	Permit intermittent denial; identify patient's primary concern

Continued

Table 6-3	Nursing Interventions for Crisis Events— cont'd
TARGET AREAS	NURSING INTERVENTIONS
Psychological Effects—cont'd	
Anxiety	Provide structure, enact antianxiety interventions
Lethargy/heroics	Encourage sublimation and constructive activity
Protective Factors	
Coping	Encourage patient's favored, adaptive coping mechanisms; emphasize rationalization, humor, sublimation
Self-efficacy	Support patient's previous successes and belief in own abilities, dilute irrational self-doubts, emphasize power of expectations to produce results
Support	Add social supports to the patient's world, provide professional support, refer for counseling when necessary, help patient develop new coping strategies

Modified from Hardin SB: Catastrophic stress. In McBride AB, Austin JK, editors: *Psychiatric–mental health nursing*, Philadelphia, 1996, WB Saunders; from US Department of Health and Human Services: *Training manual for mental health and human service workers in major disasters*, ed 2, Washington, DC, 2000, US Government Printing Office.

EVALUATION

1. Has the person returned to the precrisis level of functioning?
2. Have the person's original needs, which were threatened by the precipitating or stressful event, been met?

3. Have the person's maladaptive behaviors or symptoms subsided?
4. Have the person's adaptive coping mechanisms begun to function again?
5. Does the person have a strong support system on which to rely?
6. What has the person learned from this experience that may be helpful in coping with future crises?

 Your Internet Connection

American Institute of Stress
www.stress.org

American Red Cross
www.redcross.org/services/disaster

Crisis, Grief, and Healing
www.webhealing.com

■ REHABILITATION

Psychiatric rehabilitation is the range of social, educational, occupational, behavioral, and cognitive interventions for increasing the role performance of persons with serious and persistent mental illness and enhancing their recovery. It enables individuals to return to the highest possible level of functioning.

Psychiatric rehabilitation developed from a need to create opportunities for people diagnosed with severe mental illness to live, learn, and work in community environments of their choice. Rehabilitation proposes that those with mental illnesses should be perceived as people with disabilities. Similar to those with physical disabilities, people with psychiatric disabilities need a wide range of services, often for extended periods. Psychiatric rehabilitation uses a person-centered, people-to-people approach that differs from the traditional medical model of care (Table 7-1).

■ RECOVERY

Recovery is the process in which people are able to live, work, learn and participate fully in their communities. For some individuals, recovery is the ability to live a fulfilling and productive life, despite a disability. For others, recovery implies the reduction or complete remission of symptoms. Science has shown that **having hope** plays an integral role in an individual's recovery.

Table 7-1	Comparison of Psychiatric Rehabilitation and Traditional Medical Models of Care	
ASPECT OF CARE	PSYCHIATRIC REHABILITATION	TRADITIONAL MEDICAL REHABILITATION
Focus	Focus on wellness and health, not symptoms	Focus on disease, illness, and symptoms
Basis	Based on person's abilities and functional behavior	Based on person's disabilities and intrapsychic functioning
Setting	Caregiving in natural setting	Treatment in institutional settings
Relationship	Adult-to-adult relationship	Expert-to-patient relationship
Medication	Medicate as appropriate and tolerate some illness symptoms	Medicate until symptoms are controlled
Decision making	Case management in partnership with patient	Physician makes decisions and prescribes treatment
Emphasis	Emphasis on strengths, self-help, and interdependence	Emphasis on dependence and compliance

Characteristics of recovery as described by persons recovering from serious mental illnesses include the following (Ralph, 2000):

- *Internal factors*: factors that are within the consumer, such as awareness of the toll the illness has taken, recognition of the need to change, insight as to how this change can begin, and the determination it takes to recover
- *Self-managed care*: an extension of the internal factors in which consumers describe how they manage their own mental health and how they cope with the difficulties and barriers they face

- *External factors*: include interconnectedness with others, the supports provided by family, friends, and professionals, and having people who believe that they can cope with, and recover from, their mental illness
- *Empowerment*: a combination of internal and external factors—where internal strengths are combined with interconnectedness to provide self-help, advocacy, and caring about what happens to oneself and to others.

ASSESSMENT

The Individual

1. Identification of the nature and intensity of stressors
2. Exploration of the advantages the patient experiences by being disabled (secondary gain)
3. Identification of coping resources
4. Assessment of community living skills (Table 7-2)

The Family

1. Analysis of the family structure, including developmental stage, roles, responsibilities, norms, and values
2. Exploration of family attitudes toward the mentally ill member
3. Analysis of the emotional climate around the family
4. Identification of the social supports available to the family, including extended family, friends, financial support, religious involvement, and community contacts
5. Identification of the family's understanding of the patient's problem and the plan of care

Table 7-3 describes the categories and definitions of support needs expressed by family caregivers.

Table 7-2	Potential Skilled Activities Needed to Achieve the Goal of Psychiatric Rehabilitation		
PHYSICAL	**EMOTIONAL**	**INTELLECTUAL**

Living Skills

Personal hygiene	Human relations	Money management
Physical fitness	Self-control	Use of community
Use of public	Selective reward	resources
transportation	Stigma reduction	Goal setting
Cooking	Problem solving	Problem
Shopping	Conversational	development
Cleaning	skills	
Sports participation		
Using recreational		
facilities		

Learning Skills

Being quiet	Speech making	Reading
Paying attention	Question asking	Writing
Staying seated	Volunteering	Arithmetic
Observing	answers	Study skills
Punctuality	Following	Hobby activities
	directions	Typing
	Asking for	
	directions	
	Listening	

Working Skills

Punctuality	Job interviewing	Job qualifying
Use of job tools	Job decision	Job seeking
Job strength	making	Specific job tasks
Job transportation	Human relations	
Specific job tasks	Self-control	
	Job keeping	
	Specific job tasks	

From Anthony WA: *Principles of psychiatric rehabilitation*, Baltimore, 1908, University Park Press.

Table 7-3	Support Needs Expressed by Family Caregivers
NEED	**DESCRIPTION**

Emotional Support

Acceptance	Absence of stigmatization; acceptance of the caregiver despite his or her relationship to a mentally ill patient
Commitment	Demonstrating to the caregiver a commitment to the well-being of the patient, or sharing the burden of caregiving, if only through contact with the caregiver
Social involvement	Social contacts and companionship for the caregiver
Affective	Showing love and caring for the caregiver, including concern for his or her well-being (with qualities of sympathy, compassion, and occasionally true empathy)
Mutuality	Reciprocity in supportive exchanges

Feedback Support

Affirmation	Validation of the actions, feelings, and decisions associated with the caregiving role
Listening	Active listening by the support person, provision of a sounding board, and allowing for unburdening by the caregiver
Talking	The opportunity to talk with another person (without the quality of active listening, emotional presence, or the feeling of unburdening)

Informational or Cognitive Support

Illness information	Information about the patient's illness, care, or supervision
Behavior management	Information about behavior management strategies

Table 7-3	Support Needs Expressed by Family Caregivers—cont'd
NEED	**DESCRIPTION**

Informational or Cognitive Support —cont'd

Coping	Advice about personal coping strategies for the caregiver
Decision	Help in the decision-making process relative to caregiving issues and offering solutions
Perspective	Supportive interactions that give the caregiver a new perspective about caregiving or about the caregiving situation

Instrumental Support

Resources	Help in locating resources, negotiating systems, or advocating for needs
Respite	Provision of time off for the caregiver and support for the caregiver's own needs
Care help	Provision of help with the actual tasks of caregiving, including physical care assistance and monitoring activities (watching the patient and setting limits)
Backup	Help is available when needed, including financial help
Household	Help with such home activities as repairs, grocery shopping, and housecleaning

From Norbeck J et al: *Nurs Res* 40:208, 1991.

The Community

1. Assessment of existing community agencies that provide services to mentally ill people and their families
2. Identification of gaps in available services or in the effectiveness of existing services

Table 7-4 describes the services needed by patients with serious and persistent mental illness.

Table 7-4	Comprehensive Array of Services and Opportunities for Patients with Serious Mental Illness
BASIC NEEDS AND OPPORTUNITIES	**SPECIAL NEEDS AND OPPORTUNITIES**
Shelter	**General Medical Services**
Protected (with health, rehabilitative, or social services provided on site)	Physician assessment and care
Hospital	Nursing assessment and care
Nursing home	Dentist assessment and care
Intermediate care facility	Physical and occupational therapy
Crisis facility	Speech and hearing therapy
	Nutrition counseling
Semi-independent (linked to services)	Medication counseling
	Home health services
Family home	
Group home	**Mental Health Services**
Cooperative apartment	Acute treatment services
Foster care home	Crisis stabilization
Emergency housing facility	Diagnosis and assessment
Other board and care home	Medication monitoring (psychoactive)
	Self-medication training
Independent (access to services)	Psychotherapies
	Hospitalization: acute and long-term care
Apartment	
Home	

From Department of Health and Human Services Steering Committee on the Chronically Mentally Ill: *Toward a national plan for the chronically mentally ill*, Pub No (ADM) 81-1077, Washington, DC, 1981, US Government Printing Office.

Table 7-4	Comprehensive Array of Services and Opportunities for Patients with Serious Mental Illness—cont'd

BASIC NEEDS AND OPPORTUNITIES	SPECIAL NEEDS AND OPPORTUNITIES

Food, Clothing, and Household Management

Fully provided meals
Food purchase and preparation assistance
Access to food stamps
Homemaker service

Income or Financial Support

Access to entitlements
Employment

Meaningful Activities

Work opportunities
Recreation
Education
Religious and spiritual
Human and social interaction

Integrative Services

Patient identification and outreach
Individual assessment and service planning
Case service and resource management
Advocacy and community organization
Community information
Education and support

Habilitation and Rehabilitation

Social and recreational skills development
Life skills development
Leisure time activities

Vocational

Prevocational assessment counseling
Sheltered work opportunities
Transitional employment
Job development and placement

Social Services

Family support
Community support assistance
Housing and milieu management
Legal services
Entitlement assistance

PLANNING AND IMPLEMENTATION

The Individual

1. Mutually determine realistic nurse-patient goals based on the patient's nursing diagnoses.
2. Focus on fostering independence by maximizing the patient's strengths and potential.
3. Facilitate referrals to alternative care programs that assist the patient to function independently or interdependently in the community; may be psychosocial rehabilitation programs or community support programs.
4. Assist the patient to become involved in a social skills training program that uses cognitive and behavioral techniques.
5. Identify resistances to change, if any, and assist the patient to overcome the resistance or find acceptable alternatives.
6. Teach the patient about relevant health care needs, including physical health and mental health. This is discussed in the **Patient Education Plan related to coping with psychiatric illness** on pages 119-120.
7. Act as the patient's advocate in dealing with significant others and community agencies.
8. Assist the patient to develop a reliable social support network.

The Family

1. Establish a partnership with the family with the goal of assisting the patient.
2. Provide the patient and family with psychoeducation about the mental illness and the coping skills that will assist with successful community living (Box 7-1).
3. Provide the family with feedback on the effectiveness of their interactions.
4. Refer the family for formal family therapy if needed.
5. Refer the family to a self-help group.

PATIENT EDUCATION PLAN

COPING WITH PSYCHIATRIC ILLNESS

Content	Instructional Activities	Evaluation
Identify and describe the patient's diagnosis	Provide handouts outlining behaviors Discuss coping resources and behaviors Assign homework from lay literature Compare mental illness to physical illness	Patient recognizes characteristics of the diagnosis Patient distinguishes between cure and coping
Describe the role of stress in contributing to psychiatric disorders	Sensitize the patient to signs of increased stress Define stress as a test of coping skills Teach relaxation exercises	Patient verbalizes level of stress Patient performs relaxation exercises and describes a reduction in perceived stress
Help to gain a sense of control by recognizing personal pattern of signs and symptoms and coping strategies	Provide feedback when symptomatic behavior occurs Instruct patient to keep a diary of behavior to identify symptoms and coping strategies	Patient consistently identifies symptoms and uses an adaptive coping strategy
Enhance social and living skills to enable full participation in vocational and recreational activities	Role play social interaction in a variety of situations Review vocational preparation and current level of functioning Assess recreational activities and opportunities for future growth	Patient participates in progressively more rewarding social and work activities

Continued

PATIENT EDUCATION PLAN—CONT'D

COPING WITH PSYCHIATRIC ILLNESS

Content	Instructional Activities	Evaluation
Identify and describe community support systems	Provide a list of community support programs, including self-help groups, mental health care agencies, and social agencies Escort to first agency contact	Patient selects community programs that offer needed resources Patient becomes able to access agency independently
Describe and discuss psychoactive medications	Link the benefits of medication to the patient's personal goals Instruct about actions, side effects, and contraindications Distribute handouts describing the patient's medications Suggest systems to help patient integrate the medication regimen into the personal routine and simplify the medication schedule if possible	Patient states how medicine will help reach personal goals Patient describes characteristics of prescribed medications Patient reports effects of prescribed medications Patient takes medication as prescribed

6. Assist the family to find respite care services.
7. Provide the family with information on available crisis intervention services.

The Community

1. Provide education about mental health and mental illness to community groups.
2. Participate in community advocacy groups to encourage

BOX **7-1**

Elements of a Psychoeducation Plan

Signs and symptoms
Natural course of the illness
Possible etiologies
Diagnostic tests and measures
Indicated lifestyle changes
Treatment options
Expected treatment outcomes
Medication effects and side effects
Therapeutic strategies
Adaptive coping responses
Potential compliance problems
Early warning signs of relapse
Balancing needs and taking care of oneself

---

the development of comprehensive mental health services.

3. Foster the development of collaborative networks among community groups involved in or advocating mental health services.

4. Be aware of and involved in the political process at the local, state, and national levels.

EVALUATION

Program Evaluation

1. Individual program evaluation may include the following:
   - Cost effectiveness
   - Licensure status
   - Accomplishment of stated objectives

- Patient outcomes
- Patient, family, or staff satisfaction

2. Commonalities among a group of programs may also be assessed.
3. Programs may be evaluated at a systems level for relevance to community needs and resource utilization.

Patient Evaluation

1. The needs and levels of functioning of individual patients tend to change over time. The nurse must consider this when evaluating patient progress.
2. Evaluation criteria for individual patients must be based on the individual's behavior and treatment goals. Criteria that have been identified for evaluation of patient response to rehabilitation programs include the following:
   - Involvement in community activities, including rehabilitation programs
   - Hospitalization recidivism rates
   - Ability to find and maintain employment

◁⊙ Your Internet Connection

United States Psychiatric Rehabilitation Association
www.uspra.org

NAMI: National Alliance for the Mentally Ill
www.nami.org

New Freedom Commission on Mental Health
www.mentalhealthcommission.gov

Recovery Inc.
www.recovery-inc.com

The practice of psychiatric nursing is influenced by the law, particularly regarding the rights of patients and the quality of their care. Many of the laws vary from state to state, and nurses are required to become familiar with the legal provisions of their own state. Knowledge of the law enhances the freedom of both the nurse and the patient.

■ HOSPITALIZATION AND COMMUNITY TREATMENT

The process of hospitalization can be traumatic or supportive, depending on the institution, attitude of family and friends, response of the staff, and type of admission. Table 8-1 presents characteristics that distinguish between the two types of admission to psychiatric hospitals: voluntary and involuntary.

Involuntary Admission (Commitment)

The legal basis for involuntary confinement is either the police power of the state for the protection of society or *parens patriae*, the state's duty to protect citizens who cannot protect themselves. Figure 8-1 lists common procedural elements of the commitment process. Action is begun with a petition by a relative, friend, public official, physician, or any interested citizen stating that the person is mentally ill and in need of treatment. An examination of the patient's mental status is then completed by one or two physicians.

The decision as to whether the patient requires hospitalization is then made, and who decides this determines

Table 8-1	Characteristics of the Two Types of Admission to Psychiatric Hospitals	
	VOLUNTARY ADMISSION	**INVOLUNTARY ADMISSION**
Admission	Written application by patient	Application did not originate with patient
Discharge	Initiated by patient	Initiated by hospital or court but not by patient
Status of civil rights	Retained in full by patient	Patient may retain none, some, or all, depending on state law
Justification	Voluntarily seeks help	Mentally ill and one or more of the following: Dangerous to self or others; Needs treatment; Unable to meet own basic needs

the nature of the commitment. *Medical* certification means that physicians make the decision. *Court* or *judicial* commitment is decided by a judge or jury in a formal hearing. The patient may retain legal counsel to prepare for the hearing. *Administrative* commitment is determined by a special tribunal of hearing officers.

Most laws permit commitment of the mentally ill on the following three grounds:

1. Dangerous to self or others
2. Mentally ill and in need of treatment
3. Unable to meet basic needs such as food and shelter.

Discharge

Voluntary patients of lawful age may initiate their own discharge. Most states require that patients give written notice of their desire for discharge. For patients who are leaving

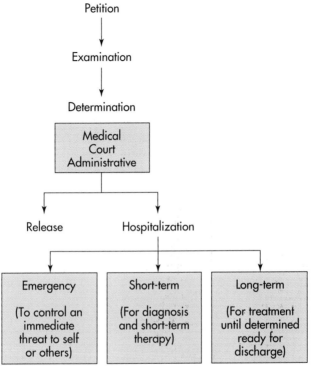

Figure 8-1 Diagram of the involuntary commitment process.

against medical advice, most hospitals request they sign a form stating this. If voluntary patients elope from the hospital, they can be brought back only if they again voluntarily agree. If they refuse to return to the hospital, they must be discharged or involuntary commitment procedures must be initiated.

Involuntary patients have lost the right to leave the hospital when they wish. If a committed patient elopes from the hospital, the staff has the legal obligation to notify the police and committing courts.

Involuntary Community Treatment

Involuntary community treatment can be provided for those in need through (1) outpatient commitment, (2) preventive commitment, and (3) conditional release from the hospital. These initiatives arose from the mandate to offer psychiatric patients treatment in the least restrictive setting.

Outpatient commitment is the process by which the courts can order patients "committed" to a course of outpatient treatment specified by their clinicians. This type of commitment provides an alternative to inpatient treatment for those who meet the involuntary commitment criterion of dangerousness to self or others.

Preventive commitment permits commitment for outpatients who do not yet meet the usual commitment criteria but will do so soon without intervention. The criteria used for preventive commitment are sometimes referred to as a *predicted deterioration standard*. In this case, a person is believed to need treatment to prevent a relapse, which would likely result in the individual becoming imminently dangerous.

Conditional release involves continued supervision of a person who has been released from the hospital. The hospital or court informs the person of the conditions for release, such as reporting to a medication clinic. Violation of these conditions usually results in rehospitalization. This approach is used primarily to determine if the individual is able to function in the community under supervision.

These initiatives are alternatives to address the pressing problem of the homeless but nondangerous mentally ill individual who is in need of psychiatric treatment and stabilization in the community. They may be most beneficial for revolving-door patients—those who stop taking their medication shortly after discharge, rapidly deteriorate, and soon require rehospitalization.

Ethical Considerations

All nurses must analyze their beliefs regarding voluntary and involuntary hospitalization and community treatment of psychiatric patients. Psychiatric nurses, patients, families, and citizens need to address such issues as the value of commitment, goals of hospitalization, treatment received while hospitalized, community alternatives, and quality of life. Nurses are responsible for reviewing commitment procedures in their state and working for the necessary clinical, ethical, and legal reforms.

■ PATIENTS' RIGHTS

Box 8-1 lists patients' rights that have been adopted by many states. Some of these rights that are especially important to psychiatric nurses are discussed next.

Right to communicate with people outside the hospital. The patient is free to visit and hold telephone conversations in privacy and send unopened letters to anyone.

Right to personal effects. The patient has the right to bring a limited number of personal items. This does not hold the hospital responsible for their safekeeping, however, and does not relieve the hospital staff of ensuring the patient's safety.

Right to execute wills. A person's competency to make a will is known as "testamentary capacity." Persons can make a valid will if they (1) know that they are making a will, (2) know the nature and extent of their property, and (3) know who their friends and relatives are and what the relationship means. Each of these criteria must be met and documented for the will to be considered valid.

Right to habeas corpus. All patients retain this right, which allows for a court of law to require the speedy release of individuals who can show they are being deprived of their liberty and detained illegally.

Right to independent psychiatric examination. The patient may demand a psychiatric examination by a physician of choice. If this physician determines that the patient is not mentally ill, the person must be released.

BOX **8-1**

Rights of Psychiatric Patients

- Right to communicate with people outside the hospital through correspondence, telephone, and personal visits
- Right to keep clothing and personal effects with them in the hospital, except for potentially dangerous objects
- Right to religious freedom
- Right to be employed, if possible
- Right to manage and dispose of property
- Right to execute wills
- Right to enter into contractual relationships
- Right to make purchases
- Right to education
- Right to habeas corpus
- Right to independent psychiatric examination
- Right to civil service status
- Right to retain licenses, privileges, or permits established by law, such as a driver's or professional license
- Right to sue or be sued
- Right to marry and divorce
- Right not to be subject to unnecessary mechanical restraints
- Right to periodic review of status
- Right to legal representation
- Right to privacy
- Right to informed consent
- Right to treatment
- Right to refuse treatment
- Right to treatment in the least restrictive setting

Right to privacy. The individual may keep some personal information completely secret from others.

Confidentiality. The principle of confidentiality allows the disclosure of certain information to another person, but this is limited to strictly authorized individuals.

Privileged communication is a legal phrase that applies only in court-related proceedings. It means that the listener cannot disclose information from an individual unless the speaker gives permission. Privileged communication does not apply to hospital charts, and most states do not provide for privileged communication between nurses and patients. In addition, therapists have the responsibility to breach the confidentiality of the relationship to warn a potential victim of impending violence by a patient.

Right to informed consent. A physician must explain the treatment to the patient, including its possible complications, side effects, and risks. The physician must obtain the patient's consent, which must be competent, understanding, and voluntary. Box 8-2 lists the reasonable information to be disclosed in obtaining informed consent.

Right to treatment. Criteria for adequate treatment are defined in three areas: (1) a humane psychological and physical environment, (2) a qualified staff with a sufficient number of members to administer treatment, and (3) individualized treatment plans.

Right to refuse treatment. Patients may refuse treatment unless they have been legally determined to be incompetent. A determination of **incompetency** requires that the person has a mental disorder resulting in a defect in judgment and that this defect makes this person incapable of handling personal affairs. Incompetency can only be reversed through another court hearing.

Ethical Considerations

Ensuring patients' rights is often complicated by ethical considerations that the nurse must carefully examine. Many ethical dilemmas arise from health care professionals' "paternalistic" attitude toward their patients, which reduces adult patients to the status of children and interferes with

BOX **8-2**

Obtaining Informed Consent

Information to Disclose
- **Diagnosis:** description of patient's problem
- **Treatment:** nature and purpose of proposed treatment
- **Consequences:** risks and benefits of proposed treatment, including physical and psychological effects, costs, and potential problems
- **Alternatives:** viable alternatives to proposed treatment and their risks and benefits
- **Prognosis:** expected outcome with treatment, with alternative treatment, and without treatment

Principles of Informing
- Assess the patient's ability to give informed consent.
- Simplify language so that laypersons can understand.
- Offer opportunities for the patient and family to ask questions.
- Test the patient's understanding after the explanation.
- Reeducate as often as needed.
- Document all relevant factors, including what was disclosed; patient's understanding, competency, and voluntary agreement to treatment; and the actual consent.

their freedom of action. Ethical questions can also arise for the psychiatric nurse when implementing patients' rights, such as the right to treatment, right to refuse treatment, and right to treatment in the least restrictive setting. All nurses participate in some therapeutic psychiatric regimens with ambiguous scientific and ethical bases. Thus each nurse must analyze such ethical dilemmas as freedom of choice versus coercion, helping versus imposing values, and focusing on cure versus prevention. Nurses assume an active role in defining adequate treatment and allocating important resources for mentally ill patients.

■ LEGISLATIVE INITIATIVES

Other legislation has also changed the nature of psychiatric care and service delivery in the United States.

Protection and Advocacy Act

Under the Protection and Advocacy for Mentally Ill Individuals Act, all states must designate an agency that is responsible for protecting the rights of mentally ill patients. The following three areas of advocacy would help to maximize the fulfillment of patients' rights:

1. Educating mental health staff and implementing policies and procedures that recognize and protect patients' rights
2. Establishing an additional procedure to permit the speedy resolution of problems, questions, or disagreements that occur based on legal rights
3. Providing access to legal services when patients' rights have been denied

Americans With Disabilities Act

The Americans with Disabilities Act (ADA), passed in 1990, protects more than 43 million people in the United States with one or more physical or mental disabilities from discrimination in jobs, public services, and accommodations. It prohibits discrimination against these persons in hiring, firing, training, compensation, and advancement in employment. Employers are prohibited from asking job applicants whether they have a disability, and medical examinations and questions about disability may be required only if the concerns are job related and necessary.

Advance Directives

Advance directives came about as a result of the Patient Self-Determination Act (PSDA) of 1990. Written while a person is competent, these documents specify how decisions about treatment should be made if the person were to become incompetent. Use of advance directives seems particularly appropriate for persons with mental illness who may alternate between periods of competence and incompetence. They could, for example, formalize a patient's wishes about forced medication or treatment setting.

■ PSYCHIATRY AND CRIMINAL RESPONSIBILITY

Three sets of criteria are used in the United States to determine the criminal responsibility of an offender with a mental illness (Table 8-2). Of these, the American Law Institute's test (ALI) is the most frequently used. The two types of insanity defense are as follows:

1. Not guilty by reason of insanity (NGBI)
2. Guilty but mentally ill (GBMI)

Both outcomes typically result in the hospitalization of patients in state mental hospitals or treatment facilities provided in a penal institution.

■ LEGAL ROLE OF THE NURSE

The psychiatric nurse has rights and responsibilities attendant to each of three legal roles: nurse as provider, nurse as employee, and nurse as citizen. Nurses may experience a conflict of interest among these rights and responsibilities. Professional nursing judgment requires a careful examination of the context of nursing care, the possible consequences of nursing actions, and the feasible alternatives the nurse might employ.

Table 8-2	Three Sets of Criteria Typically Used to Determine Criminal Responsibility of a Mentally Ill Offender

NAME OF TEST	CRITERIA
M'Naghten rule	1. The individual did not know the nature and quality of the act. 2. The individual did not know that the act was wrong.
Irresistible impulse test	An individual is impulsively driven to commit the criminal act with lack of premeditation and a strong urge to do so. This test is seldom used without other criteria.
American Law Institute's test	An individual lacks the capacity to "appreciate" the wrongfulness of the act or to "conform" conduct to the requirements of the law. It excludes the psychopath and is a popular criterion for determining criminal responsibility.

Malpractice

Malpractice involves the failure of a professional person to provide the type of care given by members of the person's profession in the community, resulting in harm to the patient. Most malpractice claims are filed under the law of *negligent tort*. A tort is a civil wrong for which the injured party is entitled to compensation. Under the law of negligent tort the plaintiff must prove the following:

1. A legal duty of care existed.
2. The nurse performed the duty negligently.
3. Damages were incurred by the patient as a result.
4. The damages were substantial.

Your Internet Connection

American Society for Bioethics and Humanities
www.asbh.org

Bazelon Center for Mental Health Law
www.bazelon.org

Medical-Legal Consulting Institute, Inc.
www.legalnurse.com

U.S. Department of Justice, Americans with Disabilities Act
www.usdoj.gov/crt/ada/adahom1.htm

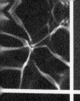

IMPLEMENTING CLINICAL PRACTICE STANDARDS

■ STANDARDS OF PSYCHIATRIC-MENTAL HEALTH CLINICAL NURSING PRACTICE

Scope and Standards of Psychiatric-Mental Health Clinical Nursing Practice describes a competent level of professional nursing care and professional performance common to nurses engaged in psychiatric-mental health nursing practice in any setting (American Nurses Association, 2000). These standards apply to nurses who are qualified by education and experience to practice at either the basic level or the advanced level of psychiatric-mental health nursing.

■ STANDARDS OF CARE*

Standards of care pertain to professional nursing activities demonstrated by the nurse throughout the nursing process. These involve assessment, nursing diagnosis, outcome identification, planning, implementation, and evaluation. The nursing process is the foundation of clinical decision making and encompasses all significant action taken by nurses in providing psychiatric-mental health care to all patients.

Figure 9-1 outlines the nursing conditions and nursing behaviors related to each of the psychiatric nursing standards of care.

---

*Reprinted with permission from American Nurses Association: Scope and standards of psychiatric-mental health clinical nursing practice, Washington, DC, 2005, The Association.

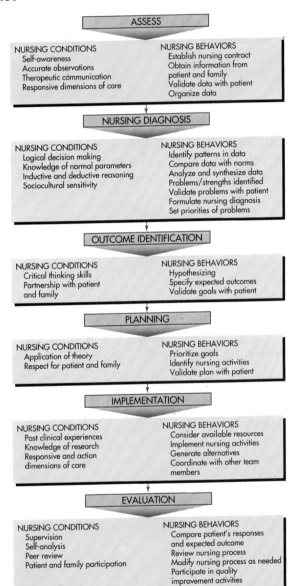

Figure 9-1 The nursing conditions and behaviors related to the psychiatric nursing standards of care.

Standard I: Assessment. The psychiatric-mental health nurse collects patient health data.

RATIONALE. The assessment interview—which requires linguistically and culturally effective communication skills, interviewing, behavior observation, database record review, and comprehensive assessment of the patient and relevant systems—enables the psychiatric-mental health nurse to make sound clinical judgments and plan appropriate interventions with the patient.

Standard II: Diagnosis. The psychiatric-mental health nurse analyzes the assessment data in determining diagnoses.

RATIONALE. The basis for providing psychiatric-mental health nursing care is the recognition and identification of patterns of response to actual or potential psychiatric illnesses and mental health problems.

Standard III: Outcome identification. The psychiatric-mental health nurse identifies expected outcomes individualized to the patient.

RATIONALE. Within the context of providing nursing care, the ultimate goal is to influence health outcomes and improve the patient's health issues.

Standard IV: Planning. The psychiatric-mental health nurse develops a plan of care that prescribes interventions to attain expected outcomes.

RATIONALE. A plan of care is used to guide therapeutic interventions systematically, document progress, and achieve the expected patient outcomes.

Standard V: Implementation. The psychiatric-mental health nurse implements the interventions identified in the plan of care.

RATIONALE. In implementing the plan of care, psychiatric-mental health nurses use a wide range of interventions designed to prevent mental and physical illness and promote, maintain, and restore mental and physical health. Psychiatric-mental health nurses select interventions according to their level of practice. At the basic level the nurse may select counseling, milieu therapy, promotion of self-care activities, intake screening and evaluation, psychobiological interventions, health teaching, case management, health promotion and health maintenance, crisis intervention, community-based care, psychiatric home health care, telehealth, and a variety of other approaches to meet the mental health needs of patients. In addition to the intervention options available to the basic-level psychiatric-mental health nurse, at the advanced level the APRN-PMH may provide consultation, engage in psychotherapy, and prescribe pharmacological agents where permitted by state statutes or regulations.

Standard Va: Counseling. The psychiatric-mental health nurse uses counseling interventions to help patients in improving or regaining their previous coping abilities, fostering mental health, and preventing mental illness and disability.

Standard Vb: Milieu therapy. The psychiatric-mental health nurse provides, structures, and maintains a therapeutic environment in collaboration with the patient and other health care providers.

Standard Vc: Self-care activities. The psychiatric-mental health nurse structures interventions around the patient's activities of daily living to foster self-care and mental and physical well-being.

Standard Vd: Psychobiological interventions. The psychiatric-mental health nurse uses knowledge of psycho-biological interventions and applies clinical skills to restore the patient's health and prevent further disability.

Standard Ve: Health teaching. The psychiatric-mental health nurse, through health teaching, assists patients in achieving satisfying, productive, and healthy patterns of living.

Standard Vf: Case management. The psychiatric-mental health nurse provides case management to coordinate comprehensive health services and ensure continuity of care.

Standard Vg: Health promotion and health maintenance. The psychiatric-mental health nurse employs strategies and interventions to promote and maintain mental health and prevent mental illness.

Advanced Practice Interventions Vh-Vj. The following interventions (Vh-Vj) may be performed only by the advanced-practice registered nurse in psychiatric-mental health nursing.

Standard Vh: Psychotherapy. The APRN-PMH uses individual, group, and family psychotherapy, child psychotherapy, and other therapeutic treatments to assist patients in preventing mental illness and disability and in improving mental health status and functional abilities.

Standard Vi: Prescription of pharmacological agents. The APRN-PMH uses prescriptive authority, procedures, and treatments in accordance with state and federal laws and regulations to treat symptoms of psychiatric illness and improve functional health status.

Standard Vj: Consultation. The APRN-PMH provides consultation to enhance the abilities of others to provide services for patients and effect change in the system.

Standard VI: Evaluation. The psychiatric-mental health nurse evaluates the patient's progress in attaining expected outcomes.

RATIONALE. Nursing care is a dynamic process involving change in the patient's health status over time, giving rise to the need for data, different diagnoses, and modifications in the plan of care. Therefore evaluation is a continuous process of appraising the effect of nursing interventions and the treatment regimen on the patient's health status and expected health outcomes.

■ STANDARDS OF PROFESSIONAL PERFORMANCE*

Standards of professional performance describe a competent level of behavior in the professional nursing role, including activities related to quality of care, performance appraisal, education, collegiality, ethics, collaboration, research, and resource utilization. All psychiatric-mental health nurses are expected to engage in professional role activities appropriate to their education, position, and practice setting. Therefore, standards or measurement criteria are used to identify these activities.

Standard I: Quality of care. The psychiatric-mental health nurse systematically evaluates the quality of care and effectiveness of psychiatric-mental health nursing practice.

RATIONALE. The dynamic nature of the mental health care environment and the growing body of psychiatric nursing knowledge and research provide both the impetus and the means for the psychiatric-mental health nurse to be competent in clinical practice, to continue to develop professionally, and to improve the quality of patient care.

Standard II: Performance appraisal. The psychiatric-mental health nurse evaluates his or her own practice in relation to professional practice standards and relevant statutes and regulations.

RATIONALE. The psychiatric-mental health nurse is accountable to the public for providing competent clinical care and has an inherent responsibility as a professional to evaluate the role and performance of psychiatric-mental health nursing practice according to standards established by the profession and regulatory bodies.

---

*Reprinted with permission from American Nurses Association: Scope and standards of psychiatric-mental health clinical nursing practice, Washington, DC, 2000, The Association.

Standard III: Education. The psychiatric-mental health nurse acquires and maintains current knowledge in nursing practice.

RATIONALE. The rapid expansion of knowledge pertaining to basic and behavioral sciences, technology, information systems, and research requires a commitment to learning throughout the psychiatric-mental health nurse's professional career. Formal education, continuing education, independent learning activities, and experiential and other learning activities are some of the means the psychiatric-mental health nurse uses to enhance nursing expertise and advance the profession.

Standard IV: Collegiality. The psychiatric-mental health nurse interacts with and contributes to the professional development of peers, health care providers, and others as colleagues.

RATIONALE. The psychiatric-mental health nurse is responsible for sharing knowledge, research, and clinical information with colleagues, through formal and informal teaching methods, to enhance professional growth.

Standard V: Ethics. The psychiatric-mental health nurse's assessments, actions, and recommendations on behalf of patients are determined and implemented in an ethical manner.

RATIONALE. The public's trust and its right to humane psychiatric-mental health care are upheld by professional nursing practice. Ethical standards describe a code of behaviors to guide professional practice. People with psychiatric-mental health needs are an especially vulnerable population. The foundation of psychiatric-mental health nursing practice is the development of a therapeutic relationship with the patient. Boundaries need to be established to safeguard the patient's well-being.

Standard VI: Collaboration. The psychiatric-mental health nurse collaborates with the patient, significant others, and health care providers in providing care.

RATIONALE. Psychiatric-mental health nursing practice requires a coordinated, ongoing interaction between consumers and providers to deliver comprehensive services to the patient and the community. Through the collaborative process, different abilities of health care providers are used to identify problems, communicate, and plan; implement interventions; and evaluate mental health services.

Standard VII: Research. The psychiatric-mental health nurse contributes to nursing and mental health through the use of research methods and findings.

RATIONALE. Nurses in psychiatric-mental health nursing are responsible for contributing to the further development of the field of mental health by participating in research. At the basic level of practice the psychiatric-mental health nurse uses research findings to improve clinical care and identifies clinical problems for research study. At the advanced level, the psychiatric-mental health nurse engages and/or collaborates with others in the research process to discover, examine, and test knowledge, theories, and creative approaches to practice.

Standard VIII: Resource Use. The psychiatric-mental health nurse considers factors related to safety, effectiveness, and cost in planning and delivering patient care.

RATIONALE. The patient is entitled to psychiatric-mental health care that is safe, effective, and affordable. As the cost of health care increases, treatment decisions must be made in such a way as to maximize resources and maintain quality of care. The psychiatric-mental health nurse seeks to provide cost-effective quality care by using the most appropriate resources and delegating care to the most appropriate, qualified health care provider.

Your Internet Connection

American Nurses Association
www.ana.org

American Psychiatric Nurses Association
www.apna.org

Canadian Nurses Association
www.cna-nurses.ca

Center for Nursing Advocacy
www.nursingadvocacy.org

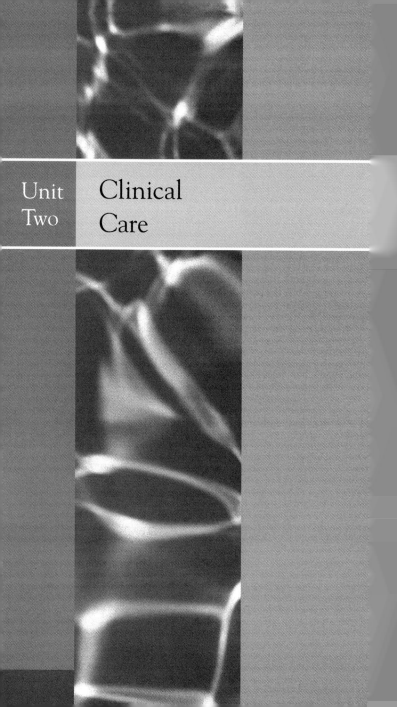

Unit
Two

Clinical
Care

■ ANXIETY RESPONSES

Anxiety is a diffuse, vague apprehension associated with feelings of uncertainty and helplessness. This emotion has no specific object. It is subjectively experienced and communicated interpersonally. It is different from **fear,** which is the intellectual appraisal of danger. Anxiety is the emotional response to that appraisal. The capacity to be anxious is necessary for survival, but severe levels of anxiety are incompatible with life. Anxiety disorders are the most common psychiatric problems in the United States.

The levels of anxiety include:

1. *Mild anxiety*—associated with the tension of daily living; it makes a person alert and increases the person's perceptual field. This anxiety can motivate learning and produce growth and creativity.

2. *Moderate anxiety*—allows a person to focus on immediate concerns and block out the periphery. It narrows the person's perceptual field. The person experiences selective inattention but can focus on more areas if directed to so do.

3. *Severe anxiety*—greatly reduces a person's perceptual field. The person tends to focus on a specific detail and not think about anything else. All behavior is aimed at obtaining relief. The person needs much direction to focus on any other area.

4. *Panic level of anxiety*—associated with awe, dread, and terror. Details are blown out of proportion. Because of

experiencing a loss of control, the person is unable to do things even with direction. Panic involves the disorganization of the personality and results in increased motor activity, decreased ability to relate to others, distorted perceptions, and loss of rational thought. This level of anxiety is incompatible with life; if it continues for a long period, exhaustion and death result.

 ASSESSMENT

Behaviors

Anxiety can be expressed directly through physiological and behavioral changes and indirectly through the formation of symptoms or coping mechanisms in an attempt to defend against anxiety. The intensity of the behaviors increases as the level of anxiety increases. Tables 10-1 and 10-2 present the physiological, behavioral, cognitive, and affective responses to anxiety.

Predisposing Factors

The following theories have been developed to explain the origins of anxiety:

1. In the *psychoanalytical* view, anxiety is the emotional conflict that takes place between two elements of the personality: the id and the superego. The id represents instinctual drives and primitive impulses, whereas the superego reflects conscience and culturally acquired restrictions. The ego, or I, serves to mediate the demands of these two opposing elements, and anxiety functions to warn the ego that it is in danger of being overtaken.

2. In the *interpersonal* view, anxiety arises from the fear of interpersonal disapproval and rejection. It is also related to developmental traumas, such as separations

Table 10-1	Physiological Responses to Anxiety	

BODY SYSTEM	RESPONSES
Cardiovascular	Palpitations
	Heart "racing"
	Increased blood pressure
	Faintness*
	Actual fainting*
	Decreased blood pressure*
	Decreased pulse rate*
Respiratory	Rapid breathing
	Shortness of breath
	Pressure on chest
	Shallow breathing
	Lump in throat
	Choking sensation
	Gasping
Neuromuscular	Increased reflexes
	Startle reaction
	Eyelid twitching
	Insomnia
	Tremors
	Rigidity
	Fidgeting, pacing
	Strained face
	Generalized weakness
	Wobbly legs
	Clumsy movement
Gastrointestinal	Loss of appetite
	Revulsion toward food
	Abdominal discomfort
	Abdominal pain*
	Nausea*
	Heartburn*
	Diarrhea*
Urinary tract	Pressure to urinate*
	Frequent urination*

*Parasympathetic response.

Table 10-1	Physiological Responses to Anxiety—cont'd	
BODY SYSTEM	**RESPONSES**	
Skin	Face flushed	
	Localized sweating (palms)	
	Itching	
	Hot and cold spells	
	Face pale	
	Generalized sweating	

Table 10-2	Behavioral, Cognitive, and Affective Responses to Anxiety	
SYSTEM	**RESPONSES**	
Behavioral	Restlessness	
	Physical tension	
	Tremors	
	Startle reaction	
	Rapid speech	
	Lack of coordination	
	Accident proneness	
	Interpersonal withdrawal	
	Inhibition	
	Flight	
	Avoidance	
	Hyperventilation	
	Hypervigilance	
Cognitive	Impaired attention	
	Poor concentration	
	Forgetfulness	
	Errors in judgment	
	Preoccupation	
	Blocking of thoughts	
	Decreased perceptual field	
	Reduced creativity	
	Diminished productivity	

Continued

Table 10-2	Behavioral, Cognitive, and Affective Responses to Anxiety—cont'd
SYSTEM	RESPONSES
Cognitive—cont'd	Confusion
	Hypervigilance
	Self-consciousness
	Loss of objectivity
	Fear of losing control
	Frightening visual images
	Fear of injury or death
	Flashbacks
	Nightmares
Affective	Edginess
	Impatience
	Uneasiness
	Tension
	Nervousness
	Fearfulness
	Alarm
	Terror
	Jitteriness
	Jumpiness
	Numbness
	Guilt
	Shame

and losses, which lead to specific vulnerabilities. People with low self-esteem are particularly vulnerable to the development of high anxiety.

3. In the *behavioral* view, anxiety is a product of frustration, which is anything that interferes with a person's ability to attain a desired goal. Other behaviorists regard anxiety as a learned drive based on an innate desire to avoid pain. Learning theorists believe that individuals who have been exposed in

early life to intense fears are more likely to be predisposed to anxiety in later life. Conflict theorists view anxiety as the clashing of two opposing interests. They believe a reciprocal relationship exists between conflict and anxiety: conflict produces anxiety, and anxiety produces feelings of helplessness, which in turn increase the perceived conflict.

4. *Family studies* show that anxiety disorders typically occur within families. Also, anxiety disorders overlap, as do anxiety disorders and depression.

5. *Biological studies* show that the brain contains specific receptors for benzodiazepines, drugs that enhance the inhibitory neuroregulator γ-aminobutyric acid (GABA), which plays a major role in biological mechanisms relating to anxiety. In addition, a person's general health and a family history of anxiety have a marked effect on predisposition to anxiety. Anxiety may accompany physical disorders and further reduce a person's capacity to cope with stressors.

Precipitating Stressors

Precipitating stressors may be derived from internal or external sources. They can be grouped into the following two categories:

1. *Threats to physical integrity* include impending physiological disability or decreased capacity to perform the activities of daily living.

2. *Threats to self-system* suggest harm to the person's identity, self-esteem, and integrated social functioning.

Coping Mechanisms

The pattern the person typically uses to cope with mild anxiety tends to remain dominant when anxiety becomes more intense. Mild levels of anxiety are often handled without conscious thought. Moderate and severe levels of anxiety elicit the following two types of coping mechanisms:

1. **Task-oriented reactions** are conscious, action-oriented attempts to meet realistically the demands of the stress situation.
   - *Attack behavior* is used to remove or overcome an obstacle to satisfy a need.
   - *Withdrawal behavior* is used to remove the self either physically or psychologically from the source of the threat.
   - *Compromise behavior* is used to change the person's usual way of operating, substitute goals, or sacrifice aspects of personal needs.
2. **Ego defense mechanisms** help to cope with mild and moderate anxiety. Because they operate on a relatively unconscious level and involve a degree of self-deception and reality distortion, however, they can be maladaptive responses to stress. Table 10-3 summarizes some of the most common ego defense mechanisms.

NURSING DIAGNOSIS

The formulation of a nursing diagnosis requires that the nurse determine the quality (appropriateness) of the patient's response, the quantity (level) of the patient's anxiety, and the adaptive or maladaptive nature of the coping mechanism used.

The box on page 158 presents the primary and related NANDA nursing diagnoses for anxiety responses. A complete nursing assessment would include all maladaptive responses of the patient. Many additional nursing problems would be identified in the way that the patient's anxiety reciprocally influenced other areas of life.

Table 10-3	Ego Defense Mechanisms	
DEFENSE MECHANISM	**DEFINITION**	**EXAMPLE**
Compensation	Process by which a person makes up for a self-image deficiency by strongly emphasizing some other feature the person regards as an asset	Mr. L, a 42-year-old businessman, perceives his small physical stature negatively. He tries to overcome this by being aggressive, forceful, and controlling in his business dealings.
Denial	Avoidance of disagreeable realities by ignoring or refusing to recognize them; probably simplest and most primitive of all defense mechanisms	Mrs. P has just been told that her breast biopsy indicates a malignancy. When her husband visits her that evening, she says that no one has discussed the laboratory results with her.
Displacement	Shift of emotion from a person or object toward which it was originally directed to another usually neutral or less dangerous person or object	Four-year-old Timmy is angry because he has just been punished by his mother for drawing on his bedroom walls. He begins to play "war" with his toy soldiers and has them fight with each other.

Continued

Table 10-3	Ego Defense Mechanisms—cont'd	
DEFENSE MECHANISM	**DEFINITION**	**EXAMPLE**
Dissociation	Separation of any group of mental or behavioral processes from the rest of consciousness or identity	A man brought to the emergency room by the police is unable to explain who he is and where he lives or works.
Identification	Process by which a person tries to become like someone the person admires by taking on the other's thoughts, mannerisms, or tastes	Sally, 15 years old, has her hair styled similarly to her young English teacher, whom she admires.
Intellectualization	Excessive reasoning or logic used to avoid experiencing disturbing feelings	A woman avoids dealing with her anxiety in shopping malls by explaining that she is saving time and money by not going into them.
Introjection	Intense type of identification in which a person incorporates qualities or values of another person or group into own ego structure; one of the earliest mechanisms of children; important in formation of conscience	Eight-year-old Jimmy tells his 3-year-old sister, "Don't scribble in your book of nursery rhymes. Just look at the pretty pictures."

Table 10-3	Ego Defense Mechanisms—cont'd	
DEFENSE MECHANISM	**DEFINITION**	**EXAMPLE**
Isolation	Splitting off of emotional components of a thought, which may be temporary or long term	A second-year medical student dissects a cadaver for her anatomy course without being disturbed by thoughts of death.
Projection	Attributing own thoughts or impulses, particularly intolerable wishes, emotional feelings, or motivations, to another person	A young woman who denies she has sexual feelings about a co-worker accuses him of trying to seduce her.
Rationalization	Offering a socially acceptable or apparently logical explanation to justify unacceptable impulses, feelings, behaviors, and motives	John fails an examination and complains that the lectures were not well organized or clearly presented.
Reaction formation	Development of conscious attitudes and behavior patterns that are opposite to what a person really feels or would like to do	A married woman who feels attracted to one of her husband's friends treats him rudely.

Continued

Table 10-3	Ego Defense Mechanisms—cont'd	
DEFENSE MECHANISM	**DEFINITION**	**EXAMPLE**
Regression	Retreat to behavior characteristic of an earlier level of development when confronted by stress	Four-year-old Nicole, who has been toilet-trained for more than a year, begins to wet her pants again when her new baby brother is brought home from the hospital.
Repression	Involuntary exclusion of a painful or conflicting thought, impulse, or memory from awareness; the primary ego defense, which other mechanisms tend to reinforce	Mr. T does not recall hitting his wife when she was pregnant.
Splitting	Viewing people and situations as either all good or all bad; failure to integrate the positive and negative qualities of the self	A friend tells you that you are the most wonderful person in the world one day, then how much she hates you the next day.
Sublimation	Acceptance of a socially approved substitute goal for a drive whose normal channel of expression is blocked	Ed has an impulsive or physically aggressive nature. He tries out for the football team and becomes a star tackle.

Table 10-3	Ego Defense Mechanisms—cont'd	
DEFENSE MECHANISM	**DEFINITION**	**EXAMPLE**
Suppression	Process often listed as a defense mechanism, but really a conscious analogue of repression; intentional exclusion of material from consciousness; at times may lead to subsequent repression	A young man at work finds he is thinking so much about his date that evening that it is interfering with his work. He decides to put it out of his mind until he leaves the office for the day.
Undoing	Act or communication that partially negates a previous one; primitive defense mechanism	Larry makes a passionate declaration of love to Sue on a date. On their next meeting he treats her formally and distantly.

Related Medical Diagnoses

Many patients experiencing transient or less severe anxiety have no medically diagnosed health problem. However, patients with more severe levels of anxiety most often have neurotic disorders that fall into the category of anxiety disorders in DSM-IV-TR.

NANDA NURSING DIAGNOSES

Related to Anxiety Responses

Adjustment, Impaired
Anxiety*
Breathing pattern, Ineffective
Communication, Impaired verbal
Confusion, Acute
Coping, Ineffective*
Coping, Readiness for enhanced*
Denial, Ineffective
Diarrhea
Fear*
Injury, Risk for
Memory, Impaired
Post-trauma syndrome
Powerlessness
Protection, Ineffective
Role performance, Ineffective
Self-esteem, Situational low
Sensory perception, Disturbed
Sleep pattern, Disturbed
Social interaction, Impaired
Thought processes, Disturbed
Tissue perfusion, Ineffective

From North American Nursing Diagnosis Association: NANDA nursing diagnoses:
definitions and classification 2005-2006, *Philadelphia, 2005, The Association.*
*Primary nursing diagnosis for anxiety.

DSM-IV-TR MEDICAL DIAGNOSES

Related to Anxiety Responses

DSM-IV-TR Diagnosis	Essential Features
Panic disorder without agoraphobia	Recurrent unexpected panic attacks (Box 10-2); at least one of the attacks has been followed by a month or more of (1) persistent concern about having additional attacks, (2) worry about the implications of the attack or its consequences, or (3) a significant change in behavior related to the attacks; also, the absence of agoraphobia.
Panic disorder with agoraphobia	Meets the above criteria plus the presence of agoraphobia, which is anxiety about being in places or situations from which escape might be difficult (or embarrassing) or in which help may not be available in the event of having an unexpected or situationally predisposed panic attack. Agoraphobic fears typically involve characteristic clusters of situations that include being outside the home alone; being in a crowd or standing in a line; being on a bridge; and traveling in a bus, train, or car. Agoraphobic situations are avoided, are endured with marked distress or with anxiety about having a panic attack, or require the presence of a companion.
Agoraphobia without history of panic disorder	Presence of agoraphobia and has never met criteria for panic disorder.

Modified from American Psychiatric Association: Diagnostic and statistical manual of mental disorders, *ed 4, text revision (DSM-IV-TR), Washington, DC, 2000, The Association.*   *Continued*

DSM-IV-TR MEDICAL DIAGNOSES

Related to Anxiety Responses—cont'd

DSM-IV-TR Diagnosis	Essential Features
Specific phobia	Marked and persistent fear that is excessive or unreasonable, cued by the presence or anticipation of a specific object or situation (e.g., flying, heights, animals, receiving an injection, seeing blood). Exposure to the phobic stimulus almost invariably provokes an immediate anxiety response. The person recognizes that the fear is excessive, and the distress or avoidance interferes with the person's normal routines.
Social phobia	Marked and persistent fear of one or more social or performance situations in which the person is exposed to unfamiliar people or to possible scrutiny by others. The individual fears that he or she will act in a way (or show anxiety symptoms) that will be humiliating or embarrassing. Exposure to the feared situation almost invariably provokes anxiety. The person recognizes that the fear is excessive, and the distress or avoidance interferes with the person's normal routine.
Obsessive-compulsive disorder	Either obsessions or compulsions (Box 10-2) are recognized as excessive and interfere with the person's normal routine.
Posttraumatic stress disorder	The person has been exposed to a traumatic event in which both the following occurred: 1. The person experienced, witnessed, or was confronted with an event or events that involved actual or threatened death or serious injury or a threat to the physical integrity of self or others.

Modified from American Psychiatric Association: Diagnostic and statistical manual of mental disorders, *ed 4, text revision (DSM-IV-TR), Washington, DC, 2000, The Association.*

DSM-IV-TR MEDICAL DIAGNOSES

Related to Anxiety Responses—cont'd

DSM-IV-TR Diagnosis	Essential Features
Posttraumatic stress disorder—cont'd	2. The person's response involved intense fear, helplessness, or horror. The person reexperiences the traumatic event, avoids stimuli associated with the trauma, and experiences a numbing of general responsiveness.
Acute stress disorder	Meets the above criteria for exposure to a traumatic event, and the person experiences three of the following symptoms: sense of detachment, reduced awareness of surroundings, derealization, depersonalization, and dissociated amnesia.
Generalized anxiety disorder	Excessive anxiety and worry, occurring more days than not for at least 6 months, about a number of events or activities. The person finds it difficult to control the worry and experiences at least three of the following six symptoms: restlessness or feeling keyed up or on edge, being easily fatigued, difficulty concentrating or mind going blank, irritability, muscle tension, and sleep disturbance.

The box on pages 159-161 describes these disorders. Criteria for panic attacks are presented in Box 10-1. Criteria for obsessions and compulsions are presented in Box 10-2.

OUTCOME IDENTIFICATION

The expected outcome for patients with maladaptive anxiety responses follows: *The patient will demonstrate adaptive ways of coping with stress.*

BOX **10-1**

Criteria for Panic Attacks

A panic attack is a discrete period of intense fear or discomfort in which at least four of the following symptoms develop abruptly and reach a peak within 10 minutes:

1. Palpitations, pounding heart, or accelerated heart rate
2. Sweating
3. Trembling or shaking
4. Sensations of shortness of breath or smothering
5. Feeling of choking
6. Chest pain or discomfort
7. Nausea or abdominal distress
8. Feeling dizzy, unsteady, lightheaded, or faint
9. Derealization (feelings of unreality) or depersonalization (being detached from self)
10. Fear of losing control or going crazy
11. Fear of dying
12. Paresthesias (numbness or tingling sensations)
13. Chills or hot flashes

PLANNING

Patients need to develop the capacity to tolerate mild anxiety and use it consciously and constructively. In this way the self becomes stronger and more integrated. A **Patient Education Plan for teaching the relaxation response** is presented on pages 164-165.

BOX 10-2

Criteria for Obsessions and Compulsions

Obsessions

Recurrent and persistent thoughts, impulses, or images are experienced at some time during the disturbance as intrusive and inappropriate and cause marked anxiety or distress.

The thoughts, impulses, or images are not simply excessive worries about real-life problems.

The person attempts to ignore or suppress such thoughts or impulses or to neutralize them with some other thought or action.

The person recognizes that the obsessional thoughts, impulses, or images are a product of his or her own mind.

Compulsions

The person feels driven to perform repetitive behaviors (e.g., handwashing, ordering, checking) or mental acts (e.g., praying, counting, repeating words silently) in response to an obsession or according to rigidly applied rules.

The behaviors or mental acts are aimed at preventing or reducing distress or preventing some dreaded event or situation; however, these behaviors or mental acts are not connected realistically with what they are designed to neutralize or prevent, or they are clearly excessive.

PATIENT EDUCATION PLAN

TEACHING THE RELAXATION RESPONSE

Content	Instructional Activities	Evaluation
Describe characteristics and benefits of relaxation.	Discuss physiological changes associated with relaxation and contrast these with anxiety behaviors.	Patient identifies own responses to anxiety. Patient describes elements of a relaxed state.
Teach deep muscle relaxation through sequence of tension-relaxation exercises.	Engage patient in progressive procedure of tensing and relaxing muscles until whole body is relaxed.	Patient can tense and relax all muscle groups. Patient identifies those muscles that become particularly tense.
Discuss relaxation procedure of meditation and its components.	Describe elements of meditation and assist patient in using this technique.	Patient selects word or scene with pleasant connotations and engages in relaxed meditation.
Assist in overcoming anxiety-provoking situations through systematic desensitization.	With patient, construct hierarchy of anxiety-provoking situations or scenes. Through imagination or reality, work through these scenes, using relaxation techniques.	Patient identifies and ranks anxiety-provoking situations. Patient exposes self to these situations while remaining relaxed.
Allow rehearsing and practical use of relaxation in a safe environment.	Have patient role-play stressful situations with you or other patients.	Patient becomes more comfortable with new behavior in a safe and supportive setting.

PATIENT EDUCATION PLAN

TEACHING THE RELAXATION RESPONSE—CONT'D

Content	Instructional Activities	Evaluation
Encourage patient to use relaxation techniques in life.	Assign use of the relaxation response in everyday experiences as homework. Support success of patient who uses relaxation in life situation.	Patient uses relaxation in real-life situations. Patient is able to regulate anxiety response through use of relaxation techniques.

 IMPLEMENTATION

Empirically validated treatments for some of the medical diagnoses related to anxiety disorders are summarized in Table 10-4.

■ INTERVENING IN SEVERE AND PANIC LEVELS OF ANXIETY

The highest-priority nursing goals should address lowering the patient's severe or panic levels of anxiety, and related nursing interventions should be supportive and protective. The **Nursing Treatment Plan Summary related to severe and panic levels of anxiety** is presented on pages 168-170.

Table 10-4	Summarizing the Evidence on Anxiety Disorders
DISORDER	**TREATMENT**
Generalized anxiety disorder (GAD)	• The most successful psychosocial treatments for GAD combine relaxation, exercise, and cognitive behavioral therapy in an effort to bring the worry process under the patient's control.
	• Benzodiazepines, buspirone, tricyclic antidepressants, venlafaxine, and selective serotonin reuptake inhibitors (SSRIs) are all effective in reducing anxiety, although the first two medications are subject to abuse/dependence.
Obsessive compulsive disorder (OCD)	• Cognitive-behavioral therapy involving exposure and ritual prevention methods reduce or eliminate the obsessions and behavioral and mental rituals of OCD.
	• Serotonin reuptake inhibitors (SRIs) reduce obsessions and compulsions in approximately 20% to 40% of cases.
Panic	• Situational in vivo exposure substantially reduces symptoms of panic disorder with agoraphobia.
	• Cognitive-behavioral treatments that focus on education about the nature of anxiety and panic provide some form of exposure, and coping skills acquisition significantly reduces symptoms of panic disorder without agoraphobia.
	• Tricyclic antidepressants and monoamine oxidase inhibitors reduce the number of panic attacks, anticipatory anxiety, and phobic avoidance.
	• The benzodiazepines eliminate panic attacks in 55% to 75% of patients.
	• SRIs and SSRIs reduce panic frequency, generalized anxiety, disability, and phobic avoidance disorder with or without agoraphobia.

ANXIETY RESPONSES AND ANXIETY DISORDERS   Chapter 10   **167**

Table 10-4	Summarizing the Evidence on Anxiety Disorders—cont'd
DISORDER	**TREATMENT**
Posttraumatic stress disorder (PTSD)	• Monoamine oxidase inhibitors (MAOIs) reduce intrusive thoughts, improve sleep, and moderate anxiety and depression. • Tricyclic antidepressants reduce intrusive thoughts and obsessions and moderate depression. • SSRIs markedly reduce intrusive thoughts, avoidance, and sleep problems. • Exposure therapies (systematic desensitization, flooding, prolonged exposure, and implosive therapy) and, to a lesser extent, anxiety management techniques (using cognitive-behavioral strategies) reduce PTSD symptoms, including anxiety and depression, and increase social functioning.
Social phobia	• Exposure-based procedures and cognitive-behavioral treatments reduce or eliminate the symptoms of the disorder. • Social skills training and relaxation techniques are effective. • MAOIs relieve the key symptoms of social phobia. • Some of the SSRIs are helpful for some aspects of the disorder.
Specific phobias	• Exposure-based procedures, especially in vivo exposure, reduce or eliminate most aspects of specific phobic disorders. • No pharmacological intervention has been shown to be effective for specific phobias.

From Nathan P, Gorman J: *A guide to treatments that work,* ed 2, New York, 2002, Oxford University Press.

/Nursing Treatment Plan Summary

Severe and Panic Anxiety Responses

Nursing Diagnosis: Severe/panic level of anxiety

Expected Outcome: Patient will reduce anxiety to a moderate or mild level.

Short-Term Goals	Interventions	Rationale
Patient will be protected from harm.	Initially accept and support, rather than attack, patient's defenses. Acknowledge reality of the pain associated with patient's present coping mechanisms. Do not focus on the phobia, ritual, or physical complaint itself. Give feedback to patient about behavior, stressors and their appraisal, and coping resources. Reinforce idea that physical health is related to emotional health and that this area will need exploration in the future. In time, begin to place limits on patient's maladaptive behavior in a supportive way.	Severe and panic levels of anxiety can be reduced by initially allowing patient to determine amount of stress that can be handled. If patient is unable to release anxiety, tension may mount to the panic level and patient may lose control. At this time, patient has no alternatives for present coping mechanisms.

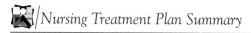

/Nursing Treatment Plan Summary

Severe and Panic Anxiety Responses—cont'd

Short-Term Goals	Interventions	Rationale
Patient will experience fewer anxiety-provoking situations.	Assume a calm manner with patient. Decrease environmental stimulation. Limit patient's interaction with other patients to minimize contagious aspects of anxiety. Identify and modify anxiety-provoking situations for patient. Administer supportive physical measures, such as warm baths and massages.	Patient's behavior may be modified by altering environment and patient's interaction with it.
Patient will engage in a daily schedule of activities.	Initially share an activity with patient to provide support and reinforce socially productive behavior. Provide for physical exercise of some type. Plan a schedule or list of activities that can be carried out daily. Involve family members and other support systems as much as possible.	By encouraging outside activities, nurse limits the time patient has available for destructive coping mechanisms while increasing participation in and enjoyment of other aspects of life.

Continued

/*Nursing Treatment Plan Summary*

Severe and Panic Anxiety Responses—cont'd

Short-Term Goals	Interventions	Rationale
Patient will experience relief from the symptoms of severe anxiety.	Administer medications that help reduce patient's discomfort. Observe for medication side effects and initiate relevant health teaching.	Effect of a therapeutic relationship may be enhanced if chemical control of symptoms allows patient to direct attention to underlying conflicts.

■ INTERVENING IN MODERATE LEVEL ANXIETY

When a patient's anxiety is reduced to the mild or moderate level, the nurse may implement insight-oriented or reeducative nursing interventions. These interventions involve the patient in a problem-solving process and are described in the Nursing Treatment Plan Summary for moderate anxiety on pages 171-173.

▧ EVALUATION

1. Have threats to the patient's physical integrity or self-system been reduced in nature, number, origin, or timing?
2. Do the patient's behaviors reflect a mild or less severe level of anxiety?
3. Have the patient's coping resources been adequately assessed and mobilized?

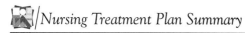

Nursing Treatment Plan Summary

Moderate Anxiety Responses

Nursing Diagnosis: Moderate level of anxiety

Expected Outcome: Patient will demonstrate adaptive ways of coping with stress.

Short-Term Goals	Interventions	Rationale
Patient will identify and describe feelings of anxiety.	Help patient identify and describe underlying feelings. Link patient's behavior with such feelings. Validate all inferences and assumptions with patient. Use open questions to move from nonthreatening topics to issues of conflict. Vary amount of anxiety to enhance patient's motivation. In time, use supportive confrontation judiciously.	To adopt new coping responses, patient first needs to be aware of feelings and to overcome conscious or unconscious denial and resistance.

Continued

/*Nursing Treatment Plan Summary*

Moderate Anxiety Responses—cont'd

Short-Term Goals	Interventions	Rationale
Patient will identify antecedents of anxiety.	Help patient describe the situations and interactions that immediately precede anxiety. Review patient's appraisal of the stressor, values being threatened, and way in which the conflict developed. Relate patient's present experiences with relevant ones from the past.	Once feelings of anxiety are recognized, patient needs to understand their development, including precipitating stressors, appraisal of the stressor, and available resources.
Patient will describe adaptive and maladaptive coping responses.	Explore how patient reduced anxiety in the past and what types of actions produced relief. Point out maladaptive and destructive effects of present coping responses. Encourage patient to use adaptive coping responses that were effective in the past. Focus responsibility for change on patient.	New adaptive coping responses can be learned through analyzing coping mechanisms used in the past, reappraising the stressor, using available resources, and accepting responsibility for change.

/Nursing Treatment Plan Summary

Moderate Anxiety Responses—cont'd

Short-Term Goals	Interventions	Rationale
	Actively help patient correlate cause-and-effect relationships while maintaining anxiety within appropriate limits.	
	Assist patient in reappraising value, nature, and meaning of the stressor when appropriate.	
Patient will implement two adaptive responses for coping with anxiety.	Help patient identify ways to restructure thoughts, modify behavior, use resources, and test new coping responses.	A person can also cope with stress by regulating the attendant emotional distress through use of stress management techniques.
	Encourage physical activity to discharge energy.	
	Include significant others as resources and social supports in helping patient learn new coping responses.	
	Teach patient relaxation exercises to increase control and self-reliance and reduce stress.	

4. Does the patient recognize his or her own anxiety and have insight into feelings?
5. Is the patient using adaptive coping responses?
6. Has the patient learned new adaptive strategies to reduce anxiety?
7. Is the patient using mild anxiety to promote personal change and growth?

🖱 Your Internet Connection

Anxiety Disorders Association of America
www.adaa.org

The Anxiety Panic Internet Resource
www.algy.com/anxiety

Freedom from Fear
www.freedomfromfear.org

National Center for PTSD
www.ncptsd.org

PSYCHOPHYSIOLOGICAL RESPONSES AND
SOMATOFORM AND SLEEP DISORDERS

■ PSYCHOPHYSIOLOGICAL RESPONSES

The degree of interconnection between mind and body has always been of interest to scientists and philosophers. In the history of medicine, body and mind were viewed for many years as separate entities. More recently, renewed attention has been given to the interrelationship between these two separate aspects of human functioning. Much of the research has focused on the stress response and the impact of stress, including the effect of psychological stress on physiological functioning, and vice versa.

ASSESSMENT

Behaviors

Many behaviors are associated with psychophysiological disorders. Careful assessment is needed to define and treat actual organic problems. This type of illness should never be dismissed as "only psychosomatic" or "all in one's head." Serious psychophysiological disorders can be fatal if not treated appropriately.

Physiological. The primary behaviors observed with psychophysiological responses are the physical symptoms. These symptoms lead the person to seek health care. Psychological factors affecting the physical condition may involve any body part. Box 11-1 lists the most common organ systems involved.

BOX 11-1

Physical Conditions Affected by Psychological Factors

Cardiovascular

Migraine
Essential hypertension
Angina
Tension headaches

Musculoskeletal

Rheumatoid arthritis
Low back pain
   (idiopathic)
Gastrointestinal
Anorexia nervosa
Peptic ulcer
Irritable bowel syndrome
Colitis
Obesity

Respiratory

Hyperventilation
Asthma

Skin

Neurodermatitis
Eczema
Psoriasis
Pruritus

Genitourinary

Impotence
Frigidity
Premenstrual syndrome

Endocrine

Hyperthyroidism
Diabetes

Psychological. Some people have physical symptoms without any organic impairment. These *somatoform disorders* include the following:

1. **Somatization disorder,** in which the person has many physical complaints
2. **Conversion disorder,** in which a loss or alteration of physical functioning occurs
3. **Hypochondriasis,** the fear or belief that the person has an illness

4. **Body dysmorphic disorder,** in which a person with a normal appearance is concerned about having a physical defect
5. **Pain disorder,** in which psychological factors play an important role in the onset, severity, or maintenance of the pain

Pain. Pain is recognized as a complex sensory and emotional experience underlying potential disease. It is influenced by behavioral, cognitive, motivational, and cultural processes and thus requires sophisticated assessments and multifaceted treatments for its control.

By definition, chronic pain consists of pain of at least 6 months' duration. *Somatoform pain disorder* is a preoccupation with pain without physical disease to account for its intensity. It does not follow a neuroanatomical distribution. A correlation also may exist between stress and conflict and the initiation or exacerbation of the pain.

Sleep. Sleep disturbances are common in the general population and among people with psychiatric disorders. Insomnia is the most prevalent sleep disorder. Up to 30% of the population have insomnia and seek help for it. Other sleep disturbances include excessive daytime sleepiness, difficulty sleeping during desired sleep time, and unusual nocturnal events such as nightmares and sleepwalking.

The consequences of sleep disorders, sleep deprivation, and sleepiness include reduced productivity, lowered cognitive performance, increased likelihood of accidents, higher risk of morbidity and mortality, and decreased quality of life. Sleep disorders are more common in elderly persons.

Sleep disorders are classified into the following four major groupings:

1. Disorders of initiating or maintaining sleep, also known as **insomnia.** Anxiety and depression are major causes of insomnia.

2. Disorders of excessive somnolence, also known as **hypersomnia.** This category includes narcolepsy, sleep apnea, and nocturnal movement disorders such as restless legs.

3. **Disorders of the sleep-wake schedule,** characterized by normal sleep but at the wrong time. These are transient disturbances often associated with jet lag and work shift changes. They are usually self-limited and resolve as the body readjusts to a new sleep-wake schedule.

4. Disorders associated with sleep stages, also known as **parasomnia.** This category includes diverse conditions such as sleepwalking, night terrors, nightmares, and enuresis. These sleep problems are often experienced by children and can have a significant effect on functioning and well-being.

Predisposing Factors

Biopsychosocial factors believed to influence the individual's psychophysiological response to stress include the following:

1. Biological factors
   - Emotions have been linked to the arousal of the neuroendocrine system through the release of corticosteroids; the actions of neurotransmitter systems; and the changes in postsynaptic receptors in response to stress.
   - Genetic factors have been shown to influence the prevalence of some psychophysiological disorders.
   - Psychoimmunology explores the connection between the mind and the immune system and is discovering biological factors that influence the way the brain protects itself from cells damaged by trauma, disease, or stress.

2. Psychological factors
   - The type A personality represents the connection of a personality type to a physiological disorder, in this case, heart disease.

- Other investigators have documented a relationship between personality style and physiological disorders such as hypertension and migraine headaches.
- Physical illness may occur with no evidence of organic impairment. In this case, psychological conflicts and anxiety are suspected to predispose a person to respond somatically.
3. Sociocultural factors
   - The severity of the person's symptoms is influenced by aspects of the social and cultural environment.
   - The symptoms shape and structure the person's social world as the illness, by its very presence, initiates a series of changes in the person's environment. The resulting chain of illness-related, interpersonal events then becomes a part of the social course of the person's illness.

Precipitating Stressors

Psychophysiological illnesses result from an attempt to cope with anxiety. The precipitating stressor may be one overwhelming experience or may seem relatively minor. Interpersonal losses are often associated with the development of physical symptoms. Sometimes a psychophysiological illness results from an accumulation of apparently minor stressful events.

Coping Mechanisms

The psychophysiological disorders may be viewed as attempts to cope with the anxiety associated with overwhelming stress. Ego defense mechanisms associated with these disorders include the following:

- Repression of feelings, conflicts, and unacceptable impulses
- Denial of psychological problems
- Compensation
- Regression

NURSING DIAGNOSIS

The individual's effort to cope with stress-related anxiety may result in numerous somatic and emotional disorders. Care must be taken to consider all the possible disruptions when formulating a complete nursing diagnosis.

The box below presents the primary and related NANDA nursing diagnoses for maladaptive psychophysiological responses. A complete nursing assessment would include all maladaptive responses of the patient, and many additional nursing diagnoses would be identified.

Related Medical Diagnoses

Medical disorders related to psychophysiological responses are classified under the general headings of somatoform disor-

---

NANDA NURSING DIAGNOSES

Related to Maladaptive Psychophysiological Responses

Adjustment, Impaired*
Anxiety
Body image, Disturbed
Coping, Ineffective
Denial, Ineffective*
Family processes, Interrupted
Health maintenance, Ineffective
Hopelessness
Pain, Chronic*
Powerlessness
Self-esteem, Situational low
Sleep pattern, Disturbed*
Spiritual distress

From North American Nursing Diagnosis Association: NANDA nursing diagnoses: definitions and classification 2005-2006, *Philadelphia, 2005, The Association.*
Primary nursing diagnosis for maladaptive psychophysiological responses.

ders, sleep disorders, and psychological factors affecting medical condition in the *DSM-IV-TR*. These are described below and on pages 182-183.

DSM-IV-TR MEDICAL DIAGNOSES

Related to Maladaptive Psychophysiological Responses

DSM-IV-TR Diagnosis	Essential Features
Somatization disorder	History of many physical complaints beginning before age 30, occurring over several years, and resulting in treatment being sought or significant impairment in social or occupational functioning. The patient must display at least four pain symptoms, two gastrointestinal symptoms, one sexual symptom, and one symptom suggesting a neurological disorder.
Conversion disorder	One or more symptoms or deficits affecting voluntary motor or sensory function and suggesting a neurological or general medical condition. Psychological factors are judged to be associated with the symptom or deficit because the initiation or exacerbation of the symptom or deficit is preceded by conflicts or other stressors. The symptom or deficit cannot be fully explained by a neurological or general medical condition and is not a culturally sanctioned behavior or experience.
Hypochondriasis	Preoccupation with fears of having, or ideas that one has, a serious disease based on the person's misinterpretation of bodily symptoms. The preoccupation persists for at least 6 months despite appropriate medical evaluation and reassurance. It causes clinically significant distress or impairment in functioning.

Continued

DSM-IV-TR MEDICAL DIAGNOSES

Related to Maladaptive Psychophysiological Responses—cont'd

DSM-IV-TR Diagnosis	*Essential Features*
Body dysmorphic disorder	Preoccupation with an imagined or exaggerated defect in appearance that causes clinically significant distress or impairment in functioning.
Pain disorder	Pain in one or more anatomical sites is predominant focus of the clinical presentation. It is of sufficient severity to warrant clinical attention and causes clinically significant distress or impairment in functioning. Psychological factors are judged to have an important role in the onset, severity, exacerbation, or maintenance of the pain.
Primary insomnia	Difficulty initiating or maintaining sleep, or nonrestorative sleep, for at least 1 month that causes clinically significant distress or impairment in functioning.
Primary hypersomnia	Excessive sleepiness for at least 1 month, as evidenced by either prolonged sleep episodes or daytime sleep episodes occurring almost daily, that causes clinically significant distress or impairment in functioning.
Narcolepsy	Irresistible attacks of refreshing sleep occurring daily over at least 3 months with cataplexy (brief episodes of sudden bilateral loss of muscle tone) and hallucinations or sleep paralysis at the beginning or end of sleep episodes.
Breathing-related sleep disorder	Sleep disruption leading to excessive sleepiness or insomnia judged to be caused by sleep apnea or central alveolar hypoventilation syndrome.

DSM-IV-TR MEDICAL DIAGNOSES

Related to Maladaptive Psychophysiological Responses—cont'd

DSM-IV-TR Diagnosis	Essential Features
Circadian rhythm sleep disorder	Persistent or recurrent pattern of sleep disruption leading to excessive sleepiness or insomnia that is caused by a mismatch between the sleep-wake schedule required by a person's environment and the circadian sleep-wake pattern and that causes clinically significant distress or impairment in functioning.
Psychological factors affecting medical condition	Presence of a medical condition in which psychological factors influence its cause, interfere with its treatment, constitute additional health risks for the individual, or elicit stress-related physiological responses that precipitate or exacerbate its symptoms.

Modified from American Psychiatric Association: Diagnostic and statistical manual of mental disorders, *ed 4, text revision (DSM-IV-TR), Washington, DC, 2000, The Association.*

OUTCOME IDENTIFICATION

The expected outcome when working with a patient with maladaptive psychophysiological responses follows:

The patient will express feelings verbally rather than through the development of physical symptoms.

PLANNING

A **Patient Education Plan for teaching adaptive coping strategies** is presented on page 184.

PATIENT EDUCATION PLAN

TEACHING ADAPTIVE COPING STRATEGIES

Content	Instructional Activities	Evaluation
Define and describe stress.	List feelings that indicate stress. Discuss behaviors associated with elevated stress.	Patient identifies behaviors associated with stressful situations.
Recognize stressful situations.	Ask patient to describe situations experienced as stressful. Role-play the situation (with videotape if possible). Discuss stress-related behaviors observed and feelings experienced.	Patient identifies stressful experiences. Patient describes own behaviors when stressed.
Review common life stressors.	Discuss common elements of stressful experiences.	Patient identifies stressful aspects of life.
Identify adaptive and maladaptive coping mechanisms.	Review the role-played stressful situations. Discuss alternative ways to cope with the stressors. Role-play at least one coping mechanism.	Patient identifies and practices adaptive coping mechanisms.
Assign use of adaptive strategy to cope with stress.	Provide feedback about effectiveness of the selected coping mechanism.	Patient selects an adaptive coping strategy when experiencing stress.

◈ IMPLEMENTATION

Empirically validated treatments for some of the medical diagnoses related to psychophysiological responses are summarized in Table 11-1.

Intervening in Psychophysiological Illness

The highest priority for nursing intervention is attending to the patient's physiological needs. This assists the patient to meet basic needs for safety and security. It is also valuable for fostering the development of a trusting relationship. Box 11-2 presents sleep hygiene strategies. A **Nursing Treatment Plan Summary for patients with maladaptive psychophysiological responses** is presented on pages 188-189.

Table 11-1	Summarizing the Evidence on Psychophysiological Responses
DISORDER	**TREATMENT**
Body dysmorphic disorder	• Cognitive-behavior therapy can help patients identify and challenge distorted body perceptions and interrupted self-critical thoughts.
Hypochondriasis	• Cognitive-behavior therapy is helpful in reducing attention to the distressing bodily sensations, correcting misinformation and exaggerated beliefs, and addressing the cognitive processes that maintain disease fears.
Pain disorder	• Individual and group cognitive-behavior therapy reduces pain-related distress and disability. • Antidepressants decrease pain intensity.

From Nathan P, Gorman J: *A guide to treatments that work*, ed 2, New York, 2002, Oxford University Press.   *Continued*

Table 11-1	Summarizing the Evidence on Psychophysiological Responses—cont'd
DISORDER	**TREATMENT**
Sleep disorders	• Benzodiazepines, zolpidem, and zaleplon reduce sleep onset by 15 to 30 minutes, decrease the number of awakenings to an absolute level of 1 to 3 per night, and increase total sleep time by about 15 to 45 minutes. These pharmacological agents act more reliably than behavioral interventions in the short term.
	• Over the long term, behavioral interventions, including stimulus control, sleep restriction, relaxation strategies, and cognitive-behavioral therapy reduce time elapsed before sleep onset, decrease awakenings, and increase total sleep time. These behavioral interventions produce more sustained effects than pharmacological agents.

EVALUATION

1. Have threats to the patient's physical integrity or self-system been reduced in nature, origin, or timing?
2. Do the patient's behaviors reflect greater self-awareness and acceptance of emotional experiences?
3. Have the patient's coping resources been adequately assessed and mobilized?
4. Does the patient recognize the level of stress, and does the patient have insight into own feelings?
5. Is the patient using adaptive coping responses?

BOX **11-2**

Sleep Hygiene Strategies

- Set a regular bedtime and wake-up time 7 days a week.
- Exercise daily to aid sleep initiation and maintenance; however, vigorous exercise too close to bedtime may make falling asleep difficult.
- Schedule time to wind down and relax before bed.
- Avoid worrying when trying to fall asleep.
- Guard against nighttime interruptions. Earplugs may help with a noisy partner. Heavy window shades help to screen out light. Create a comfortable bed.
- Maintain a cool temperature in the room. A warm bath or warm drink before bed helps some people fall asleep.
- Excessive hunger or fullness may interfere with sleep. Avoid large meals before bed. If hungry, a light carbohydrate snack may be helpful.
- Avoid caffeinated drinks, excessive fluid intake, stimulating drugs, and excessive alcohol in the evening and before bedtime.
- Excessive napping may make it difficult for some people to fall asleep at night.
- Do not eat, read, work, or watch television in bed. The bed and bedroom should be used only for sleep and sex.
- Maintain a reasonable weight. Excessive weight may result in daytime fatigue and sleep apnea.
- Get out of bed and engage in other activities if not able to fall asleep.

6. Has the patient learned new adaptive strategies to cope effectively with life stressors?
7. Is the patient using greater self-understanding to promote personal change and growth?

▧/Nursing Treatment Plan Summary

Maladaptive Psychophysiological Responses

Nursing Diagnosis: Impaired adjustment

Expected Outcome: Patient will express feelings verbally rather than through the development of physical symptoms.

Short-Term Goals	Interventions	Rationale
Patient will identify areas of stress and conflict and relate feelings, thoughts, and behaviors to them.	Assist patient in identifying stressful situations by reviewing events surrounding the development of physical symptoms. Facilitate the association among thoughts, feelings, and behaviors.	Inability to deal with intrapsychic conflict leads to anxiety and stress, resulting in physiological dysfunction.
Patient will describe present defenses and evaluate whether they are adaptive or maladaptive.	Proceed slowly in analyzing defenses. Explore alternative coping behaviors with patient. Teach patient stress management techniques (e.g., relaxation, imagery).	Defenses should not be attacked; rather, nurse should support positive exploration of patient and suggest alternative responses.

/*Nursing Treatment Plan Summary*

Maladaptive Psychophysiological Responses—cont'd

Short-Term Goals	Interventions	Rationale
Patient will adopt two new coping mechanisms to deal with stress.	Give patient positive feedback for new adaptive behaviors. Actively support patient in testing new coping mechanisms. Enlist support of family and significant others to reinforce change.	Change requires time and positive reinforcement from others. Family members can be particularly important in promoting adaptive responses.
Patient will display decreased physical symptoms and greater biological integrity.	Encourage physical activity to reduce stress. Counsel patient on diet and nutrition needs. Review patient's sleep habits and promote good sleep hygiene practices.	Wellness requires a balance between biological and psychosocial needs. Interventions focused on patient's physiological needs can help patient restore biological integrity.

✎ Your Internet Connection

Academy of Psychosomatic Medicine
www.apm.org

American Pain Foundation
www.painfoundation.org

American Pain Society
www.ampainsoc.org

American Psychosomatic Society
www.psychosomatic.org

American Academy of Sleep Medicine
www.aasmnet.org

National Sleep Foundation
www.sleepfoundation.org

The Sleep Medicine Home Page
www.users.cloud9.net/~thorpy

The SLEEP WELL
www.stanford.edu/~dement

12 | SELF-CONCEPT RESPONSES AND DISSOCIATIVE DISORDERS

■ SELF-CONCEPT RESPONSES

Self-concept is defined as all the notions, beliefs, and convictions that constitute an individual's knowledge of self and that influence relationships with others. Self-concept does not exist at birth; it is learned as a result of a person's unique experiences within the self, with significant others, and with worldly realities.

Self-concept consists of the following components:

1. **Body image**—the sum of the individual's conscious and unconscious attitudes toward his or her body. It includes present and past perceptions and feelings about size, function, appearance, and potential. Body image is modified continually by new perceptions and experiences.
2. **Self-ideal**—the individual's perception of how he or she should behave based on certain personal standards, aspirations, goals, or values.
3. **Self-esteem**—the individual's judgment of personal worth obtained by analyzing how well one's behavior conforms to self-ideal. High self-esteem is a feeling rooted in unconditional acceptance of self, despite mistakes, defeats, and failures, as an innately worthy and important being.
4. **Role performance**—sets of socially expected behavior patterns associated with an individual's function in various social groups. *Ascribed roles* are assigned roles over which the person has no choice. *Assumed roles* are those selected or chosen by the individual.

5. **Personal identity**—the organizing principle of the personality that accounts for the individual's unity, continuity, consistency, and uniqueness. It connotes autonomy and includes perceptions of one's sexuality. Identity formation begins in infancy and proceeds throughout life but is the major task of the adolescent period.

An individual with a **healthy personality** experiences the following:

- Positive and accurate body image
- Realistic self-ideal
- Positive self-concept
- High self-esteem
- Satisfying role performance
- Clear sense of identity

Identity diffusion is an individual's failure to integrate various childhood identifications into a harmonious adult psychosocial personality. **Depersonalization** is a feeling of unreality and alienation from the self. It is associated with the panic level of anxiety and failure in reality testing. The individual has difficulty distinguishing the self from others, and the person's body has an unreal and strange quality about it.

ASSESSMENT

Behaviors

Data collection by the nurse should include both objective and observable behaviors and the patient's subjective and internal world. Boxes 12-1 to 12-3 list behaviors related to low self-esteem, identity diffusion, and depersonalization.

Predisposing Factors

Numerous factors contribute to alterations in an individual's self-concept. These include factors affecting the following:

BOX **12-1**

Behaviors Associated With Low Self-Esteem

- Criticism of self and others
- Decreased productivity
- Destructiveness toward others
- Disruptions in relatedness
- Exaggerated sense of self-importance
- Feelings of inadequacy
- Guilt
- Irritability or excessive anger
- Negative feelings about one's body
- Perceived role strain
- Pessimistic view of life
- Physical complaints
- Polarizing view of life
- Rejection of personal capabilities
- Self-destructiveness
- Self-diminution
- Social withdrawal
- Substance abuse
- Withdrawal from reality
- Worrying

1. *Self-esteem* including parental rejection, unrealistic parental expectations, repeated failures, lack of personal responsibility, dependency on others, and unrealistic self-ideals.
2. *Role performance* including gender role stereotypes, work role demands, and cultural role expectations.
3. *Personal identity* including parental distrust, peer pressure, and changes in the social structure.

Precipitating Stressors

Precipitating stressors may be derived from internal or external sources as follows:

BOX **12-2**

Behaviors Associated With Identity Diffusion

- Absence of moral code
- Contradictory personality traits
- Exploitative interpersonal relationships
- Feelings of emptiness
- Fluctuating feelings about self
- Gender confusion
- High degree of anxiety
- Inability to empathize with others
- Lack of authenticity
- Problems with intimacy

BOX **12-3**

Behaviors Associated With Depersonalization

Affective

Feelings of alienation from self
Feelings of insecurity, inferiority, shame
Feelings of unreality
Heightened sense of isolation
Inability to derive pleasure or sense of accomplishment
Lack of sense of inner continuity
Loss of identity

Perceptual

Auditory and visual hallucinations
Confusion about one's sexuality
Difficulty distinguishing self from others
Disturbed body image
Experiencing world as dreamlike

1. *Trauma* such as sexual and psychological abuse or witnessing a life-threatening event
2. *Role strain* associated with expected roles or positions that the person experiences as frustration; the three types of role transitions follow:
   - *Developmental role transitions* are normative changes associated with growth. They include developmental stages in an individual's or family's life and cultural norms, values, and pressures to conform.
   - *Situational role transitions* occur with the addition or subtraction of significant others through birth or death.
   - *Health-illness role transitions* result from moving from a well state to an illness state. Such transitions may be precipitated by the following:
     - Loss of a body part
     - Changes in body size, shape, appearance, or function
     - Physical changes associated with normal growth and development
     - Medical and nursing procedures

Coping Mechanisms

Coping mechanisms include short-term or long-term coping defenses and the use of ego defense mechanisms to protect the person from facing painful self-perceptions.

Short-term defenses include the following:

1. Activities that provide temporary escape from the person's identity crisis (e.g., loud rock concerts, hard physical labor, obsessive television watching)
2. Activities that provide temporary substitute identities (e.g., joining social, religious, or political clubs, groups, movements, or gangs)
3. Activities that serve temporarily to strengthen or heighten a diffuse sense of self (e.g., competitive sports, academic achievement, popularity contests)

   4. Activities that represent short-term attempts to make
      an identity out of the meaninglessness of life itself
      (e.g., drug abuse)

Long-term defenses include the following:
   1. *Identity foreclosure*—the premature adoption of an
      identity that is desired by significant others without
      coming to terms with one's own desires, aspirations,
      or potential
   2. *Negative identity*—assumption of an identity that is at
      odds with accepted values and accepted expectations
      of society

Ego defense mechanisms include the use of fantasy, dissociation, isolation, projection, displacement, splitting, turning
anger against self, and acting out.

NURSING DIAGNOSIS

Problems with self-concept are associated with feelings of
anxiety, hostility, and guilt. These often create a circular and
self-propagating process for the individual that ultimately
results in maladaptive coping responses. These responses can
be seen in a variety of people experiencing threats to their
physical integrity or self-system.

   The box on page 197 presents the primary and related
NANDA nursing diagnoses for maladaptive self-concept
responses. A complete nursing assessment would include all
maladaptive responses of the patient. Many additional nursing problems would be identified in the way that the patient's
self-concept reciprocally influenced other areas of life.

Related Medical Diagnoses

Because they pertain to a person's basic personality structure
and feelings about the self, the nursing diagnoses related to
self-concept can include a variety of medical disorders. A

NANDA NURSING DIAGNOSES

Related to Maladaptive Self-Concept Responses

Anxiety
Body image, Disturbed*
Communication, Impaired verbal
Coping, Ineffective
Hopelessness
Identity, Disturbed personal*
Impaired religiosity, Risk for
Powerlessness
Role performance, Ineffective*
Self-concept, Readiness for enhanced*
Self-esteem, Chronic low, Situational low, Risk for situational low*
Sexuality pattern, Ineffective
Social interaction, Impaired
Spiritual distress
Spiritual distress, Risk for
Thought processes, Disturbed

From North American Nursing Diagnosis Association: NANDA nursing diagnoses: definitions and classification 2005-2006, *Philadelphia, 2005, The Association.*
Primary nursing diagnosis for alterations in self-concept.

number of specific medical diagnoses have dominant features that relate to one's self-concept. The box on page 198 identifies and describes these diagnoses.

OUTCOME IDENTIFICATION

The expected outcome when working with a patient with a maladaptive self-concept response follows:
The patient will obtain the maximum level of self-actualization to realize one's potential.

DSM-IV-TR MEDICAL DIAGNOSES

Related to Maladaptive Self-Concept Responses

DSM-IV-TR Diagnosis	Essential Features
Identity problem	Uncertainty about multiple issues relating to identity, such as long-term goals, career choice, friendship patterns, sexual orientation and behavior, moral values, and group loyalties.
Dissociative amnesia	Predominant disturbance is one or more episodes of inability to recall important personal information, usually of a traumatic or stressful nature, that is too extensive to be explained by ordinary forgetfulness.
Dissociative fugue	Predominant disturbance is sudden, unexpected travel away from home or one's customary place of work, with inability to recall one's past. Confusion about personal identity or assumption of a new identity.
Dissociative identity disorder (multiple personality disorder)	Presence of two or more distinct identities or personality states (each with its own relatively enduring pattern of perceiving, relating to, and thinking about the environment and self). At least two of these identities or personality states recurrently take control of the person's behavior. Inability to recall important personal information that is too extensive to be explained by ordinary forgetfulness.
Depersonalization disorder	Persistent or recurrent experiences of feeling detached from and as if one is an outside observer of one's mental processes or body (e.g., feeling as if one is in a dream). During the depersonalization experience, reality testing remains intact. The depersonalization causes clinically significant distress or impairment in functioning.

Modified from American Psychiatric Association: Diagnostic and statistical manual of mental disorders, *ed 4, text revision (DSM-IV-TR), Washington, DC, 2000, The Association.*

PLANNING

A **Patient Education Plan for improving family relationships** is presented below and on page 200.

 PATIENT EDUCATION PLAN

IMPROVING FAMILY RELATIONSHIPS

Content	Instructional Activities	Evaluation
Define concept of self-differentiation in a person's family of origin.	Discuss differences between high and low levels of self-differentiation. Ask patient to identify level of functioning among family members.	Patient identifies own functioning level in family of origin.
Describe characteristics of emotional fusion, emotional cutoff, and triangulation.	Analyze types and patterns of family relationships.	Patient describes interactional patterns in own family.
	Use paper and pencil to diagram family patterns.	Patient identifies own roles and behavior.
Discuss role of symptom formation and symptom bearer in a family.	Sensitize patient to family dynamics and manifestations of stress.	Patient recognizes family's contribution to stress of individual members.
	Encourage family communication.	Patient contacts family members.

Continued

PATIENT EDUCATION PLAN

IMPROVING FAMILY RELATIONSHIPS—CONT'D

Content	Instructional Activities	Evaluation
Describe a family genogram and show how it is constructed.	Use a blackboard to map out a family genogram.	Patient obtains factual information about family.
	Assign family genogram.	Patient constructs family genogram.
Analyze need for objectivity and responsibility for changing own behavior and not that of others.	Role-play interactions with various family members.	Patient demonstrates higher level of differentiation in family of origin.
	Encourage testing out new ways of interacting with family members.	

 IMPLEMENTATION

Empirically validated treatments for one of the medical disorders related to self-concept responses are summarized in Table 12-1.

Intervening in Alterations in Self-Concept

Nursing intervention helps the patient examine his or her cognitive appraisal of the situation and related feelings to

Table 12-1	Summarizing the Evidence on Treatments that Work for Self-Concept Responses
DISORDER	TREATMENT
Dissociative disorders	• Sodium pentobarbital, sodium amobarbital, and hypnosis are useful in facilitating the recovery of repressed and dissociated memories. • Psychotherapy helps patients work through and ultimately control access to traumatic memories.

From Nathan P, Gorman J: *A guide to treatments that work,* ed 2, New York, 2002, Oxford University Press.

help the patient gain insight and then take action to bring about behavioral change. This problem-solving approach requires progressive levels of intervention as follows:

1. Expanded self-awareness
2. Self-exploration
3. Self-evaluation
4. Realistic planning
5. Commitment to action

Tables 12-2 through 12-6 describe specific principles, rationales, and nursing interventions for each progressive level in the sequence. A **Nursing Treatment Plan Summary for maladaptive self-concept responses** is presented on page 211-213.

EVALUATION

1. Have threats to the patient's physical integrity or self-system been reduced in nature, number, origin, or timing?

Table 12-2	Nursing Interventions for Alterations in Self-Concept at Level 1	
PRINCIPLE	**RATIONALE**	**NURSING INTERVENTIONS**

Goal: To Expand Patient's Self-Awareness

Establish an open, trusting relationship.	Reduce threat that nurse poses to patient; help patient to broaden and accept all aspects of personality.	Offer unconditional acceptance. Listen to patient. Encourage discussion of patient's thoughts and feelings. Respond nonjudgmentally. Convey that patient is a valued person who is responsible for and able to help self.
Work with whatever ego strength patient possesses.	Some degree of ego strength, such as capacity for reality testing, self-control, or a degree of ego integration, is needed as a foundation for later nursing care.	Identify patient's ego strength. Use guidelines for patient with limited ego resources: 1. Begin by confirming patient's identity. 2. Provide support measures to reduce panic level of anxiety. 3. Approach patient in nondemanding way. 4. Accept and attempt to clarify any verbal or nonverbal communication. 5. Prevent patient from isolating self. 6. Establish simple routine for patient. 7. Set limits on inappropriate behavior.

Table 12-2	Nursing Interventions for Alterations in Self-Concept at Level 1—cont'd	
PRINCIPLE	**RATIONALE**	**NURSING INTERVENTIONS**
		8. Orient patient to reality.
		9. Reinforce appropriate behavior.
		10. Gradually increase activities and tasks that provide positive experiences.
		11. Assist in personal hygiene and grooming.
		12. Encourage patient in self-care.
Maximize patient's participation in therapeutic relationship.	Mutuality is necessary for patient to assume ultimate responsibility for own behavior and maladaptive coping responses.	Gradually increase patient's participation in care decisions. Convey that patient is a responsible individual.

Table 12-3	Nursing Interventions for Alterations in Self-Concept at Level 2	
PRINCIPLE	**RATIONALE**	**NURSING INTERVENTIONS**
Goal: To Expand Patient's Self-Exploration		
Assist patient to accept own feelings and thoughts.	By showing interest in and accepting patient's feelings and thoughts, nurse helps patient to do the same.	Attend to and encourage patient's expression of emotions, beliefs, behavior, and thoughts—verbally, nonverbally, symbolically, or directly. Use therapeutic communication skills and empathic responses. Note patient's use of logical and illogical thinking and reported and observed emotional responses.
Help patient clarify concept of self and relationship to others through self-disclosure.	Self-disclosure and understanding self-perceptions are prerequisites to bringing about future change; this alone may reduce anxiety.	Elicit patient's perception of self-strengths and weaknesses. Assist patient to describe self-ideal. Identify patient's self-criticisms. Help patient to describe beliefs on how he or she relates to other people and events.

Table 12-3	Nursing Interventions for Alterations in Self-Concept at Level 2—cont'd	
PRINCIPLE	**RATIONALE**	**NURSING INTERVENTIONS**
Be aware of and have control of own feelings.	Self-awareness allows nurse to model authentic behavior and limits potential negative effects of countertransference in relationship.	Be open to own feelings. Accept both positive and negative feelings. Practice therapeutic use of self: 1. Share own feelings with patient. 2. Verbalize how another might have felt. 3. Mirror own perception of patient's feelings.
Respond empathically, not sympathetically, emphasizing that power to change lies with patient.	Sympathy can reinforce patient's self-pity; rather, nurse should communicate that patient's life situation is subject to self-control.	Use empathic responses and monitor self for feelings of sympathy or pity. Reaffirm that patient is not helpless or powerless in face of problems. Convey verbally and behaviorally that patient is responsible for own behavior, including choice of maladaptive or adaptive coping responses. Discuss scope of patient's choices, areas of ego strength, and available coping resources.

Continued

Table 12-3	Nursing Interventions for Alterations in Self-Concept at Level 2—cont'd	
PRINCIPLE	RATIONALE	NURSING INTERVENTIONS
		Use support systems of family and groups to facilitate patient's self-exploration. Assist patient in recognizing nature of conflict and maladaptive coping responses.

Table 12-4	Nursing Interventions for Alterations in Self-Concept at Level 3	
PRINCIPLE	RATIONALE	NURSING INTERVENTIONS

Goal: To Expand Patient's Self-Evaluation

| Help patient define the problem clearly. | Only after problem is accurately defined can alternative choices be proposed. | Identify relevant stressors and patient's appraisal of them. Clarify that patient's beliefs influence both feelings and behaviors. Mutually identify faulty beliefs, misperceptions, distortions, illusions, and unrealistic goals. Mutually identify areas of strength. Place concepts of success and failure in proper perspective. Explore patient's use of coping resources. |

Table 12-4	Nursing Interventions for Alterations in Self-Concept at Level 3—cont'd	
PRINCIPLE	**RATIONALE**	**NURSING INTERVENTIONS**
Explore patient's adaptive and maladaptive coping responses to the problem.	It is necessary to examine patient's coping choices and evaluate both positive and negative consequences.	Describe to patient how all coping responses are freely chosen and have both positive and negative consequences. Contrast adaptive and maladaptive responses. Mutually identify disadvantages of patient's maladaptive coping responses. Mutually identify advantages, or "payoffs," of patient's maladaptive coping responses. Discuss how these payoffs have perpetuated the maladaptive response. Use variety of therapeutic skills, such as: 1. Facilitative communication 2. Supportive confrontation 3. Role clarification 4. Transference and countertransference reaction in the one-to-one relationship 5. Psychodrama

Table 12-5	Nursing Interventions for Alterations in Self-Concept at Level 4	
PRINCIPLE	**RATIONALE**	**NURSING INTERVENTIONS**
Goal: To Assist Patient in Formulating a Realistic Plan of Action		
Help patient identify alternative solutions.	Only when all possible alternatives have been evaluated can change be effected.	Help patient understand that only he or she can change self, not others. If patient holds inconsistent perceptions, help patient see how to change the following: 1. Beliefs or ideals to bring them closer to reality 2. Environment to make it consistent with patient's beliefs If self-concept is not consistent with behavior, help patient see how to change the following: 1. Behavior to conform to self-concept 2. Beliefs underlying self-concept to include behavior 3. Self-ideal Mutually review how patient may better use coping resources.

Table 12-5	Nursing Interventions for Alterations in Self-Concept at Level 4—cont'd	
PRINCIPLE	RATIONALE	NURSING INTERVENTIONS
Help patient conceptualize own realistic goals.	Goal setting must include a clear definition of the expected change.	Encourage patient to formulate own (not nurse's) goals. Mutually discuss emotional, practical, and reality-based consequences of each goal. Help patient clearly define the concrete change to be made. Encourage patient to enter new experiences for their growth potential. Use role rehearsal, role modeling, role playing, and visualization when appropriate.

2. Do the patient's behaviors reflect greater self-acceptance, self-worth, and self-approval?
3. Have the patient's coping resources been adequately assessed and mobilized?
4. Has the patient expanded self-awareness and engaged in self-exploration and self-evaluation?
5. Is the patient using adaptive coping responses?
6. Has the patient learned new adaptive strategies to enhance the level of self-actualization?
7. Is the patient using greater self-understanding to promote personal change and growth?

Table 12-6	Nursing Interventions for Alterations in Self-Concept at Level 5	
PRINCIPLE	**RATIONALE**	**NURSING INTERVENTIONS**

Goal: To Assist Patient to Become Committed to Decision and Achieve Own Goals

PRINCIPLE	RATIONALE	NURSING INTERVENTIONS
Help patient take necessary action to change maladaptive coping responses and maintain adaptive ones.	Ultimate objective in promoting insights is to have patient replace maladaptive coping responses with more adaptive ones.	Provide opportunity for patient to experience success. Reinforce strengths, skills, and healthy aspects of patient's personality. Help patient gain assistance (vocational, financial, social services). Use groups to enhance patient's self-esteem. Promote patient's self-differentiation in family of origin. Allow patient sufficient time to change. Provide appropriate amount of support and positive reinforcement to help patient maintain progress.

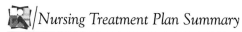
/Nursing Treatment Plan Summary

Maladaptive Self-Concept Responses

Nursing Diagnosis: Self-esteem disturbance

Expected Outcome: Patient will obtain the maximal level of self-actualization to realize his or her potential.

Short-Term Goals	Interventions	Rationale
Patient will establish a therapeutic relationship with nurse.	Confirm patient's identity. Provide supportive measures to decrease panic level of anxiety. Set limits on inappropriate behavior. Work with whatever ego strengths patient possesses. Reinforce adaptive behavior.	Mutuality is necessary for patient to assume responsibility for behavior. Some degree of ego integrity is needed for later interventions.
Patient will express feelings behaviors, and thoughts related to present stressful situations.	Assist patient to express and describe feelings and thoughts. Help patient in identifying strengths and weaknesses, self-ideal, and self-criticisms. Respond empathically, emphasizing that the power to change lies within patient.	Self-disclosure and understanding are necessary to bring about change. Use of sympathy is not therapeutic because it can reinforce patient's self-pity; rather, nurse should communicate that patient is in control.

Continued

/*Nursing Treatment Plan Summary*

Maladaptive Self-Concept Responses—cont'd

Short-Term Goals	Interventions	Rationale
Patient will evaluate the positive and negative consequences of self-concept responses.	Identify relevant stressors and patient's appraisal of them. Clarify faulty beliefs and cognitive distortions. Evaluate advantages and disadvantages of current coping responses.	Only after the problem is defined can alternative choices be examined; then the positive and negative consequences of current patterns must be evaluated.
Patient will identify one new goal and two adaptive coping responses.	Encourage patient to formulate a new goal. Help patient clearly define the change to be made. Use role rehearsal, role modeling, and visualization to practice the new behavior.	Only after alternatives have been explored can change be effected. Goal setting specifies nature of the change and suggests possible new behavioral strategies.

/Nursing Treatment Plan Summary

Maladaptive Self-Concept Responses—cont'd

Short-Term Goals	Interventions	Rationale
Patient will implement the new adaptive self-concept responses.	Provide opportunity for patient to experience success. Reinforce strengths, skills, and adaptive coping responses. Allow patient sufficient time to change. Promote group and family involvement. Provide appropriate amount of support and positive reinforcement for patient to maintain progress and growth.	Ultimate goal in promoting patient's insight is to have patient replace the maladaptive coping responses with more adaptive ones.

 Your Internet Connection

International Society for the Study of Dissociation
www.issd.org

National Association for Self-Esteem
www.self-esteem-nase.org

Self-Esteem Learning Foundation
www.selfesteem.org

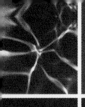

■ EMOTIONAL RESPONSES

Mood refers to a prolonged emotional state that influences an individual's whole personality and life functioning. It pertains to a person's prevailing and pervading emotion and is synonymous with the terms *affect*, *feeling state*, and *emotion*. As with other aspects of the personality, emotions or moods serve an adaptive role for the individual. Emotional responses include:

1. **Emotional responsiveness**—being affected by and being an active participant in one's internal and external worlds; being open to and aware of one's feelings.

2. **Uncomplicated grief reaction**—a response to a loss in which the person is facing the reality of the loss and is immersed in the work of grieving.

3. **Suppression of emotions**—the denial of one's feelings, a detachment from them, or an internalization of all aspects of one's affective world.

4. **Delayed grief reaction**—the persistent absence of any emotional response to a loss. The delay may occur at the start of the mourning process, may become evident later in the process, or both.

5. **Depression**—an abnormal extension or overelaboration of sadness and grief; used to denote a variety of phenomena, such as a sign, symptom, syndrome, emotional state, reaction, disease, or clinical entity.

6. **Mania**—characterized by an elevated, expansive, or irritable mood. *Hypomania* is used to describe a

clinical syndrome similar to but not as severe as that described by the term *mania* or *manic* episode.

Box 13-1 presents facts about depressive and bipolar (manic-depressive) disorders.

BOX **13-1**

Facts About Mood Disorders

Major Depressive Disorder

- Major depression is among the most common of all clinical problems encountered by primary care practitioners.
- Major depression accounts for more bed days (people off work and in bed) than any other "physical" disorder except cardiovascular disease. Depression is more costly to the economy than chronic respiratory illness, diabetes, arthritis, or hypertension.
- Psychotherapy alone helps some depressed patients, especially those with mild to moderate symptoms.
- Depression can be treated successfully with antidepressant medications in 65% of patients.
- Treatment success rates increase to 85% when alternative or adjunctive medications are used or psychotherapy is combined with medications.

Bipolar (Manic-Depressive) Disorder

- Without modern treatments, patients with bipolar disorder typically spend one fourth of their adult life in the hospital and half of their life disabled.
- Effective medications (lithium, anticonvulsants), often used in combination with supportive psychotherapy, allow 75% to 80% of manic-depressive patients to lead essentially normal lives.
- These drugs have saved the U.S. economy more than $40 billion since 1970: $13 billion in direct treatment costs and $27 billion in indirect costs.

ASSESSMENT

Behaviors

The behaviors associated with depression are varied (Box 13-2). Sadness and slowness may predominate, or states of agitation may occur. The key element to a behavioral assessment is change—the individual **changes the usual behavioral pattern and responses**.

BOX **13-2**

Behaviors Associated With Depression	
Affective	Loss of interest and motivation
Anger	Pessimism
Anxiety	Self-blame
Apathy	Self-deprecation
Bitterness	Self-destructive thoughts
Dejection	Uncertainty
Denial of feelings	
Despondency	**Physiological**
Guilt	Abdominal pain
Helplessness	Anorexia
Hopelessness	Backache
Loneliness	Chest pain
Low self-esteem	Constipation
Sadness	Dizziness
Sense of worthlessness	Fatigue
	Headache
Cognitive	Impotence
Ambivalence	Indigestion
Confusion	Insomnia
Inability to concentrate	Lassitude
Indecisiveness	

Continued

BOX **13-2**

Behaviors Associated With Depression—cont'd

Physiological—cont'd

Menstrual changes
Nausea
Overeating
Sexual nonresponsiveness
Sleep disturbances
Vomiting
Weight change

Behavioral

Aggressiveness
Agitation
Alcoholism

Altered activity level
Drug addiction
Intolerance
Irritability
Lack of spontaneity
Overdependency
Poor personal hygiene
Psychomotor retardation
Social isolation
Tearfulness
Underachievement
Withdrawal

The essential feature of mania is a distinct period of intense psychophysiological activation. Box 13-3 lists some behaviors associated with mania.

Predisposing Factors

Various theories have been proposed to explain severe disturbances of mood. The range of causative factors, which may operate singly or in combination, is evident in the following theories and models:

1. *Genetic factors* have been proposed to account for the transmission of affective disorders through heredity and family history.
2. *Aggression-turned-inward theory* suggests that depression results from the turning of angry feelings inward against the self.
3. *Object loss theory* refers to the traumatic separation of a person from significant objects of attachment.

BOX **13-3**

Behaviors Associated With Mania

Affective
Elation or euphoria
Expansiveness
Humor
Inflated self-esteem
Intolerance of criticism
Lack of shame or guilt

Cognitive
Ambition
Denial of realistic danger
Distractibility
Flight of ideas
Grandiosity
Illusions
Lack of judgment
Loose associations

Physiological
Dehydration
Inadequate nutrition

Need for little sleep
Weight loss

Behavioral
Aggression
Excessive spending of
  money
Grandiose acts
Hyperactivity
Increased motor activity
Irresponsibility
Irritability or
  argumentativeness
Poor personal grooming
Provocation
Sexual overactivity
Social activity
Verbosity

4. *Personality organization theory* describes how a negative self-concept and low self-esteem influence a person's belief system and appraisal of stressors.
5. *Cognitive model* proposes that depression is a cognitive problem dominated by one's negative evaluation of oneself, one's world, and one's future.
6. *Learned helplessness model* suggests that trauma per se does not produce depression, but rather the belief that one has no control over the important outcomes in one's life; therefore the person refrains from making adaptive responses.

7. *Behavioral model* is derived from the social learning theory framework, which assumes the cause of depression resides in the individual's lack of positively reinforcing interactions with the environment.

8. *Biological model* describes the chemical changes in the body that occur during depressed states, including the deficiency of catecholamines, endocrine dysfunction, hypersecretion of cortisol, neurotransmitter dysregulation, and periodic variations in biological rhythms.

Precipitating Stressors

Four major sources of stressors can precipitate a disturbance of mood as follows:

1. *Loss of attachment,* real or imagined, includes the loss of love, a person, physical functioning, status, or self-esteem. Because of the actual and symbolic elements involved in the concept of loss, the patient's perceptions take on primary importance.

2. *Major life events* frequently precede a depressive episode and affect a person's current problems and problem-solving abilities.

3. *Role strain* contributes to the development of depression, particularly in women.

4. *Physiological changes* produced by drugs or various physical illnesses (e.g., infections, neoplasms, metabolic imbalances) can precipitate disturbances of mood. Various antihypertensive drugs and the abuse of addictive substances are common precipitating factors. Most chronic, debilitating illnesses are also frequently accompanied by depression. Depression in elderly persons is particularly complex because the diagnosis often involves evaluating for organic brain damage and clinical depression.

Box 13-4 lists the risk factors for depression.

BOX **13-4**

Risk Factors for Depression
Prior episodes of depression
Family history of depression
Prior suicide attempts
Female gender
Age of onset less than 40 years
Postpartum period
Medical comorbidity
Lack of social support
Stressful life events
Personal history of sexual abuse
Current substance abuse

Coping Mechanisms

A delayed grief reaction reflects the exaggerated use of the defense mechanisms of denial and suppression in an attempt to avoid the intense distress associated with grief. Depression is similar to abortive grieving, using the mechanisms of repression, suppression, denial, and dissociation. Some believe that mania is a mirror image of depression and that, even though the behaviors are dissimilar, the dynamics and coping mechanisms are related.

NURSING DIAGNOSIS

The diagnosis of mood disturbance depends on an understanding of many interrelated concepts, including anxiety, self-concept, and hostility. The box on page 221 presents the primary and related NANDA nursing diagnoses for maladaptive emotional responses.

NANDA NURSING DIAGNOSES

Related to Maladaptive Emotional Responses

Anxiety
Communication, Impaired verbal
Coping, Ineffective
Grieving, Anticipatory
Grieving, Dysfunctional*
Grieving, Risk for dysfunctional
Hopelessness*
Powerlessness*
Self-esteem, Chronic low or Situational low
Sexual dysfunction
Sleep pattern, Disturbed
Social isolation
Spiritual distress*
Spiritual distress, Risk for
Suicide, Risk for*
Violence, Risk for self-directed*

From North American Nursing Diagnosis Association: NANDA nursing diagnoses:
definitions and classification 2005-2006, *Philadelphia, 2005, The Association.*
*Primary nursing diagnoses for disturbances in mood.

Related Medical Diagnoses

The two major categories of mood or affective disorders identified in DSM-IV-TR, bipolar (manic-depressive) disorders and depressive (unipolar) disorders, are based on whether manic and depressive episodes are present over time.

In the **depressive disorder** classification, major depression may involve either a single episode or a recurrent depressive illness but without manic attacks. When the patient has one or more manic episodes, with or without a major depressive episode, the category of **bipolar disorder** is used. The box on pages 222-223 describes medical diagnoses related to mood disorders. Box 13-5 lists diagnostic criteria for major depressive and manic episodes.

DSM-IV-TR MEDICAL DIAGNOSES

Related to Maladaptive Emotional Responses

DSM-IV-TR Diagnosis	*Essential Features*
Bipolar I disorder	Current or past experience of a manic episode, lasting at least 1 week, when the person's mood was abnormally and persistently elevated, expansive, or irritable. The episode is sufficiently severe to cause extreme impairment in social or occupational functioning. Bipolar disorders may be classified as manic (limited to only manic episodes), depressed (history of manic episodes with a current depressive episode), or mixed (both manic and depressive episodes).
Bipolar II disorder	Presence or history of one or more major depressive episodes and at least one hypomanic episode. The person has never had a manic episode.
Cyclothymic disorder	History of 2 years of hypomania in which the person experienced numerous periods with abnormally elevated, expansive, or irritable moods. These moods did not meet the criteria for a manic episode, and many periods of depressed mood did not meet the criteria of a major depressive episode.
Major depressive disorder	Presence of at least five symptoms during the same 2-week period, with one being either depressed mood or loss of interest or pleasure. Other symptoms might include weight loss, insomnia, psychomotor agitation or retardation, fatigue, feelings of worthlessness, diminished ability to think, and recurrent thoughts of death. Major depressions may be classified as a single episode or recurrent.

Modified from American Psychiatric Association: Diagnostic and statistical manual of mental disorders, *ed 4, text revision (DSM-IV-TR), Washington, DC, 2000, The Association.*   *Continued*

DSM-IV-TR MEDICAL DIAGNOSES

Related to Maladaptive Emotional Responses—cont'd

DSM-IV-TR Diagnosis	*Essential Features*
Dysthymic disorder	At least 2 years of a usually depressed mood and at least one of the symptoms mentioned for major depression without meeting the criteria for a major depressive episode.

BOX **13-5**

Diagnostic Criteria for Major Depressive and Manic Disorders

Major Depressive Episode

At least five of the following (including one of the first two) must be present most of the day, almost daily, for at least 2 weeks.

1. **Depressed mood**
2. **Loss of interest or pleasure**
3. Weight loss or gain
4. Insomnia or hypersomnia
5. Psychomotor agitation or retardation
6. Fatigue or loss of energy
7. Feelings of worthlessness
8. Impaired concentration
9. Thoughts of death or suicide

Manic Episode

At least three of the following must be present to a significant degree for at least 1 week.

1. Grandiosity
2. Decreased need for sleep
3. Pressured speech
4. Flight of ideas
5. Distractibility
6. Psychomotor agitation
7. Excessive involvement in pleasurable activities without regard for negative consequences

OUTCOME IDENTIFICATION

The expected outcome when working with a patient with a maladaptive emotional response follows:

The patient will be emotionally responsive and return to pre-illness level of functioning.

PLANNING

In care planning, the nurse's priorities are the reduction and ultimate removal of all the patient's maladaptive emotional responses, restoration of the patient's occupational and psychosocial functioning, improvement in the patient's quality of life, and minimization of the likelihood of relapse and recurrence. To achieve this, treatment consists of three phases: (1) acute, (2) continuation, and (3) maintenance (Figure 13-1).

Acute

The goal of acute treatment is to produce a **response,** which is the elimination of the symptoms. A successful acute phase treatment brings patients back to an essentially

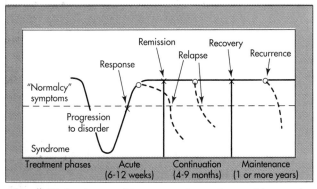

Figure 13-1 Phases of treatment for patients with mood disorders.

symptom-free state and to a level of functioning comparable to that before the illness. This phase usually lasts **6 to 12 weeks,** and if patients are symptom free at the end of that time, they are in **remission**.

Continuation

The goal of continuation treatment is to prevent **relapse,** which is the return of symptoms. The risk of relapse is very high in the first 4 to 6 months after recovery, and one of the greatest mistakes in the treatment of mood disorders is the failure to continue a successful treatment for sufficient time. This phase usually lasts **4 to 9 months.**

Maintenance

The goal of maintenance treatment is to prevent the **recurrence,** or return, of a new episode of illness. This concept is commonly accepted for bipolar illness but is relatively new for major depressive disorders. Several research studies indicate the effectiveness of maintenance therapy in preventing new depressive episodes or lengthening the interval between them.

A **Patient Education Plan for enhancing social skills** is presented on page 226.

IMPLEMENTATION

Empirically validated treatments for major depressive disorder and bipolar disorder are summarized in Table 13-1.

Intervening in Depression and Mania

Nursing interventions must reflect the complex nature of the integrative model of mood disturbances and address all maladaptive aspects of a patient's life. Intervening in as many areas as possible should have the greatest effect. A **Nursing Treatment Plan Summary** for patients with maladaptive emotional responses begins on page 229.

PATIENT EDUCATION PLAN

ENHANCING SOCIAL SKILLS

Content	Instructional Activities	Evaluation
Describe behaviors interfering with social interactions.	Instruct patient on corrective behaviors.	Patient identifies problematic and more facilitative behaviors.
Discuss components of social performance relevant to patient's situation.	Model effective interpersonal skills for patient.	Patient describes specific skills to acquire.
Analyze how patient could incorporate these specific skills.	Use role playing and guided practice to allow patient to test new behaviors.	Patient shows beginning skill in new social behaviors.
Encourage patient to test new skills in other situations.	Give homework assignments for patient to do in natural environment.	Patient discusses ability to complete assigned tasks.
Discuss generalization of new skills to other aspects of patient's life and functioning.	Give feedback, encouragement, and praise for newly acquired social skills and their generalization.	Patient is able to integrate new social behaviors in interactions with others.

Table 13-1	Summarizing the Evidence on Mood Disorders

DISORDER	TREATMENT
Major depressive disorder (MDD)	• Interventions using behavior therapy, cognitive-behavior therapy, and interpersonal therapy are all effective treatments. • Because of their narrow safety margin and significant drug-induced adverse side effects, tricyclic antidepressants (TCAs) have now been largely replaced for the treatment of depression by selective serotonin reuptake inhibitors (SSRIs), including fluoxetine, sertraline, paroxetine, and citalopram, along with newer compounds such as venlafaxine, mirtazapine, bupropion, and nefazodone. • One large study supports the superior effectiveness of combined psychosocial and pharmacological treatment. • Because of adverse side effects, monoamine oxidase inhibitors (MAOIs) are generally reserved for treatment-refractory MDD patients.
Bipolar disorder	• Lithium, divalproex and olanzapine are all effective in reducing the symptoms of acute bipolar manic episodes. • Carbamazepine; typical antipsychotics, risperidone and ziprasidone, are effective in the treatment of acute mania.

From Nathan P, Gorman J: *A guide to treatments that work*, ed 2, New York, 2002, Oxford University Press.

Table 13-1	Summarizing the Evidence on Mood Disorders–cont'd
DISORDER	**TREATMENT**
Bipolar disorder—cont'd	• Although understudied, the pharmacological treatment of acute bipolar depression suggests that lithium, most antidepressants, and lamotrigine are effective antidepressants.
	• Lithium is effective with many patients in preventing or reducing the frequency of recurrent affective episodes, although side effects have been a problem with drug adherence.
	• Divalproex and carbamazepine are effective preventive treatments.
	• Although pharmacological interventions are treatments of choice, psychosocial treatments, including psychoeducation, cognitive-behavioral therapy, interpersonal therapy, and marital/family therapy help to increase medication adherence, improve quality of life, and enhance coping mechanisms of patients with bipolar disorder.

/*Nursing Treatment Plan Summary*

Maladaptive Emotional Responses

Nursing Diagnosis: Hopelessness

Expected Outcome: Patient will be emotionally responsive and return to pre-illness level of functioning.

Short-Term Goals	Interventions	Rationale
Patient's environment will be safe and protective.	Continually evaluate patient's potential for suicide. Hospitalize patient at risk for suicide. Assist patient to move to a new environment when appropriate (e.g., new job, peer group, family setting).	All patients with severe mood disturbances are at high risk for suicide; environmental changes can protect patient, decrease immediate stress, and mobilize additional resources.
Patient will establish a therapeutic relationship with nurse.	Use a warm, accepting, empathic approach. Be aware of and in control of own feelings and reactions (e.g., anger, frustration, sympathy). *With depressed patient:* Establish rapport through shared time and supportive companionship. Allow patient time to respond.	Both depressed and manic patients resist becoming involved in a therapeutic alliance; acceptance, persistence, and limit setting are necessary.

/*Nursing Treatment Plan Summary*

Maladaptive Emotional Responses—cont'd

Short-Term Goals	Interventions	Rationale
	Personalize care as a way of indicating patient's value as a human being. *With manic patient:* Give simple, truthful responses. Be alert to possible manipulation. Set constructive limits on negative behavior. Use a consistent approach by all health team members. Maintain open communication and sharing of perceptions among team members. Reinforce patient's self-control and positive aspects of patient behavior.	
Patient will be physiologically stable and able to meet self-care needs.	Assist patient to meet self-care needs, particularly in areas of nutrition, sleep, and personal hygiene. Encourage patient's independence whenever possible. Administer prescribed medications and somatic treatments.	Physiological changes occur with disturbances of mood; physical care and somatic therapies are required to overcome these problems.

Continued

/*Nursing Treatment Plan Summary*

Maladaptive Emotional Responses—cont'd

Short-Term Goals	Interventions	Rationale
Patient will be able to recognize and express emotions related to daily events.	Respond empathically with a focus on feelings rather than facts. Acknowledge patient's pain and convey a sense of hope in recovery. Help patient experience feelings and then express them appropriately. Assist patient in adaptive expression of anger.	Patients with severe mood disturbances have difficulty identifying, expressing, and modulating feelings.
Patient will evaluate thinking and correct faulty or negative thoughts.	Review patient's conceptualization of the problem but do not necessarily accept conclusions. Identify patient's negative thoughts and help decrease them. Help increase positive thinking. Examine the accuracy of perceptions, logic, and conclusions. Identify misperceptions, distortions, and irrational beliefs.	These strategies help increase patient's sense of control over goals and behaviors, enhance self-esteem, and modify negative expectations.

/*Nursing Treatment Plan Summary*

Maladaptive Emotional Responses—cont'd

Short-Term Goals	Interventions	Rationale
Patient will implement two new behavioral coping strategies.	Help patient move from unrealistic to realistic goals. Decrease importance of unattainable goals. Limit amount of patient's negative personal evaluations. Assign appropriate action-oriented therapeutic tasks. Encourage activities gradually, escalating them as patient's energy is mobilized. Provide a tangible, structured program when appropriate. Set goals that are realistic, relevant to patient's needs and interests, and focused on positive activities. Focus on present activities, not past or future activities. Positively reinforce successful performance. Incorporate physical exercise in patient's plan of care.	Successful behavioral performance counteracts feelings of helplessness and hopelessness.

Continued

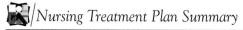/*Nursing Treatment Plan Summary*

Maladaptive Emotional Responses—cont'd

Short-Term Goals	Interventions	Rationale
Patient will describe rewarding social interactions.	Assess patient's social skills, supports, and interests. Review existing and potential social resources. Instruct and model effective social skills. Use role playing and rehearsal of social interactions. Give feedback and positive reinforcement of effective interpersonal skills. Intervene with families to have them reinforce patient's adaptive emotional responses. Support or engage in family and group therapy when appropriate.	Socialization is an experience incompatible with withdrawal and increases self-esteem through the social reinforcers of approval, acceptance, recognition, and support.

♩ NURSE **ALERT**

In caring for the patient with a severe mood disorder, the nurse should give highest priority to the potential for suicide. Hospitalization is definitely indicated for the patient at risk for suicide. In the presence of rapidly progressing symptoms and in the absence or rupture of the usual support systems, hospitalization is strongly indicated. Nursing care in this case means protecting patients and assuring them that they will not be allowed to harm themselves. Patients are at particular risk for suicide when they appear to be coming out of depression; they may then have the energy and opportunity to commit suicide. Acute manic states are also life threatening.

EVALUATION

1. Were all possible sources of precipitating stress and the patient's perception of them explored?
2. Was the patient appropriately assessed for problems related to self-concept, anger, and interpersonal relationships?
3. Were changes in the patient's usual behavioral patterns and responses explored?
4. Was the patient's personal and family history of previous episodes of depression or elation fully evaluated?
5. Were appropriate precautions taken for possible suicide or self-harm?
6. Was the patient's social network supported as a coping resource?
7. Were the nursing interventions broad in scope and inclusive of the many aspects of the patient's world?
8. Were the patient's transference reactions identified and worked through?

9. Was the nurse aware of personal feelings, conflicts, and ability to confront the range of emotions openly throughout the therapeutic relationship?
10. Is the patient experiencing increased satisfaction and pleasure?

Your Internet Connection

Bipolar Disorders Portal
www.pendulum.org

Depression and Bipolar Support Alliance
www.dbsalliance.org

Depression and Related Affective Disorders Association
www.drada.org

Depression Screening
www.depression-screening.org

Dr. Ivan's Depression Central
www.psycom.net/depression.central.html

National Alliance for Research on Schizophrenia and Depression
www.narsad.org

National Foundation for Depressive Illness, Inc.
www.depression.org

■ SELF-PROTECTIVE RESPONSES

Self-destructive behavior is any activity that will lead to death if not interrupted. It may be classified as direct or indirect. **Direct self-destructive behavior** includes any form of suicidal activity. The intent is death, and the individual is aware of this as the desired outcome. The behavior is short term in duration. **Indirect self-destructive behavior** includes any activity that is detrimental to a person's physical well-being and that can lead to death. The person is unaware of this potential and usually denies it if confronted. The behavior is usually longer in duration than suicidal behavior. Indirect self-destructive behaviors include the following:

- Cigarette smoking
- Reckless driving
- Gambling
- Criminal activity
- Participation in high-risk recreational activities
- Substance abuse
- Socially deviant behavior
- Stress-seeking behavior
- Eating disorders
- Noncompliance with medical treatment

ASSESSMENT

Behaviors

Noncompliance. It has been estimated that one half of patients do not comply with their health care treatment plan. People who do not comply with recommended health care activities are generally aware that they have chosen not to care for themselves. Box 14-1 lists the most prominent behaviors associated with noncompliance.

Self-Injury. Various terms have been used to describe self-injurious behavior: *self-abuse, self-directed aggression, self-harm, self-inflicted injury,* and *self-mutilation.* Self-injury can be defined as the act of deliberately harming one's own body. The injury is done to oneself, without the aid of another person, and the injury is severe enough for tissue damage. Common forms of self-injurious behavior include cutting and burning the skin, banging the head and limbs, picking at wounds, and chewing fingers.

BOX **14-1**

Behaviors Associated With Treatment Noncompliance

Awareness of a reason for noncompliance
Minimization of the seriousness of the problem
Chronic illnesses characterized by asymptomatic intervals
Frequent changes in health care providers
Search for miracle cures
Guilt that interferes with obtaining regular care
Concern about control

Suicidal Behavior. All suicidal behavior is serious, what-
ever the intent. In the assessment of suicidal behavior, much
emphasis is placed on the lethality of the method threatened
or used. Although all suicide threats and attempts must be
taken seriously, more vigorous and vigilant attention is indicated when the person is planning or tries a highly lethal
means, such as a gunshot, hanging, or jumping. Less lethal
means include carbon monoxide and drug overdose, which
allow time for discovery once the suicidal action has begun.
Assessment of the suicidal person also includes whether the
person has made a specific plan and whether the means to
carry out the plan are available.

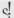 **NURSE ALERT**

> The most suicidal person is one who plans a violent death,
> has a specific plan, and has the means readily available.

Suicidal behavior is usually divided into the following three
categories:
1. *Suicide threats*—verbal or nonverbal warnings that a
   person is considering suicide. Suicidal persons may
   indicate verbally that they will not be around much
   longer or may communicate nonverbally by giving
   away prized possessions, revising a will, and so on.
   These messages should be considered in the context
   of current life events. The threat represents the
   person's ambivalence about dying. Lack of a positive
   response may be interpreted as encouragement to
   carry out the act.
2. *Suicide attempts*—any self-directed actions taken by
   the individual that will lead to death if not
   interrupted.

3. *Completed suicide*—may take place after warning signs have been missed or ignored. Persons who make suicide attempts and who do not really intend to die may do so if they are not discovered in time.

♂ NURSE **ALERT**

Directly questioning the patient about suicidal thought and plans will not result in the patient taking suicidal actions. Rather, most people feel relieved to be asked about these feelings. One of the most important questions to ask suicidal patients is whether they think they can control their behavior and refrain from acting on their impulses. If they cannot do this, immediate psychiatric hospitalization is indicated.

Predisposing Factors

Five domains of predisposing factors contribute to understanding self-destructive behavior over the life cycle:

1. *Psychiatric diagnosis*—more than 90% of adults who end their lives by suicide have an associated psychiatric illness. Three psychiatric disorders that put individuals at particular risk for suicide are mood disorders, substance abuse, and schizophrenia.
2. *Personality traits*—the three aspects of personality that are most closely associated with increased risk of suicide are hostility, impulsivity, and depression.
3. *Psychosocial milieu*—recent bereavement, separation or divorce, early loss, and decreased social supports are important factors related to suicide.
4. *Family history*—a family history of suicide is a significant risk factor for self-destructive behavior.
5. *Biochemical factors*—data suggest that serotonin-, opiate-, and dopamine-mediated processes may be implicated in self-destructive behavior.

Precipitating Stressors

Self-destructive behavior may result from almost any stress the individual feels is overwhelming. Precipitants are often humiliating life events, such as interpersonal problems, public embarrassment, loss of a job, or threat of incarceration. In addition, knowing someone who attempted or committed suicide or being exposed to suicide through the media may also make the individual more vulnerable to self-destructive behavior. Box 14-2 lists factors that the nurse must consider in the assessment of a self-destructive patient.

BOX **14-2**

Factors in the Assessment of the Self-Destructive Patient

Circumstances of an Attempt
Precipitating humiliating life event
Preparatory actions: acquiring a method, putting affairs in order, suicidal talk, giving away prized possessions, suicidal note
Use of violent method or more lethal drugs/poisons
Understanding of lethality of chosen method
Precautions taken against discovery

Presenting Symptoms
Hopelessness
Self-reproach, feelings of failure and unworthiness
Depressed mood
Agitation and restlessness
Persistent insomnia
Weight loss
Slowed speech, fatigue, social withdrawal
Suicidal thoughts and plans

BOX **14-2**

Factors in the Assessment of the
Self-Destructive Patient—cont'd

Psychiatric Illness
Previous suicide attempt
Mood disorders
Alcoholism or substance abuse
Conduct disorders and depression in adolescents
Early dementia and confusional states in elderly
    schizophrenia
Combinations of the above

Psychosocial History
Recently separated, divorced, or bereaved
Living alone
Unemployed, recent job change or loss
Multiple life stresses (move, early loss, breakup of
    important relationship, school problems, threat of
    disciplinary crisis)
Chronic medical illness
Excessive drinking or substance abuse

Personality Factors
Impulsivity, aggressivity, hostility
Cognitive rigidity and negativity
Hopelessness
Low self-esteem
Borderline or antisocial disorder

Family History
Family history of suicidal behavior
Family history of mood disorder, alcoholism, or both

BOX 14-3

Suicide Risk Factors

Psychosocial and Clinical
Hopelessness
Caucasian race
Male gender
Advanced age
Living alone

History
Prior suicide attempts
Family history of suicide attempts
Family history of substance abuse

Diagnostic
General medical illness
Psychosis
Substance abuse
Mood disorders

Although it is not possible to predict suicide, the nurse must assess each individual for known suicide risk factors (Box 14-3) and determine the meaning of each of these elements for potential suicidal behavior.

Coping Mechanisms

Ego defense mechanisms related to indirect self-destructive behavior are (1) denial, the most prominent coping mechanism; (2) rationalization; (3) intellectualization; and (4) regression. Defense mechanisms should not be challenged without offering alternative means of coping. They may be standing between the person and suicide.

Suicidal behavior indicates the imminent failure of the coping mechanisms. A suicidal threat may be one last effort to obtain sufficient help to be able to cope. Completed suicide represents the failure of the coping and adaptive mechanisms.

NURSING DIAGNOSIS

The diagnosis of self-destructive behavior must be based on consideration of the seriousness and immediacy of the patient's harmful activity. Patient denial of the self-destructive nature of the behavior must not be allowed to persuade the nurse to underestimate the need for nursing intervention.

The nursing diagnosis is related to the nurse's observations combined with data collected by other health care providers and the information provided by the patient and significant others. The box below presents the primary and related NANDA nursing diagnoses for maladaptive self-protective responses.

NANDA NURSING DIAGNOSES

Related to Maladaptive Self-Protective Responses

Adjustment, Impaired
Anxiety
Coping, Ineffective
Denial, Ineffective
Hopelessness
Noncompliance*
Powerlessness
Self-esteem, Chronic low or Situational low
Self-mutilation*
Spiritual distress
Spiritual distress, Risk for
Suicide, Risk for*
Violence, Risk for self-directed*

From North American Nursing Diagnosis Association: NANDA nursing diagnoses: definitions and classification 2005-2006, *Philadelphia, 2005, The Association.*
*Primary nursing diagnosis for self-destructive behavior.

Related Medical Diagnoses

Several medical diagnostic classifications include actual or potential self-destructive behavior among the defining criteria. Suicidal behavior is not separately identified as a diagnostic category. Therefore this section includes medical diagnoses in which this type of behavior is listed as possible. The disorders included in this section are described in the DSM-IV-TR and are identified in the box below.

DSM-IV-TR MEDICAL DIAGNOSES

Related to Self-Protective Responses

DSM-IV-TR Diagnosis	Essential Features
Bipolar disorder	Presence of a manic episode and no past depressive episodes (see Chapter 13).
Major depressive disorder	Presence of at least five symptoms almost daily during the same 2-week period, with one being either depressed mood or loss of interest or pleasure (see Chapter 13).
Noncompliance with treatment	Noncompliance with an important aspect of treatment for a mental disorder or a general medical condition.
Schizophrenia	Presence of two or more of the following symptoms for a 1-month period: delusions, hallucinations, disorganized speech, disorganized behavior, and negative symptoms (see Chapter 15).
Substance use disorders	Presence of substance dependence or substance abuse (see Chapter 18).

Modified from American Psychiatric Association: Diagnostic and statistical manual of mental disorders, *ed 4, text revision (DSM-IV-TR), Washington, DC, 2000, The Association.*

OUTCOME IDENTIFICATION

The expected outcome when working with a patient with maladaptive self-protection responses is as follows:

The patient will not inflict physical self-injury.

PLANNING

The nursing care plan for the person with self-destructive behavior must focus first on protecting the patient from harm. In addition, the plan must address the factors that contributed to the patient's dangerous behavior. The planning process also involves providing the patient with education about the specific illness. A **Patient Education Plan on compliance counseling for a patient with a medical treatment** is presented below and on page 246.

 PATIENT EDUCATION PLAN

COMPLIANCE COUNSELING

Content	Instructional Activities	Evaluation
Assess patient's knowledge of self-care activities.	Ask patient to describe usual lifestyle, diet, exercise, and medication patterns.	Patient describes usual behavior.
	Do described behaviors match self-care instruction received in the past?	Patient repeats previous directions.
Identify areas in which patient behavior differs from healthy self-care practices.	Describe healthy self-care behavior to patient. Provide written patient education materials. Encourage patient to describe reasons for not performing recommended self-care.	Patient discusses problems with compliance.
Discuss alternative approaches to self-care.	Assist patient to identify alternative and more acceptable self-care behaviors.	Patient decides on different approach, shares feelings related to illness.

PATIENT EDUCATION PLAN

COMPLIANCE COUNSELING—CONT'D

Content	Instructional Activities	Evaluation
	Enable patient to talk about feelings related to illness and treatment.	
Agree on a reward for compliant behavior.	Ask patient about reward for practicing good self-care.	Patient identifies reward.
Reinforce new behavior.	Praise patient for making commitment to healthier lifestyle.	Patient recognizes renewed commitment to self-care. ,

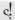 NURSE **ALERT**

Patients identified as suicidal require special attention from the nurse, who should remember the following guidelines:

1. Take all threats of suicide, verbal or nonverbal, seriously. Report them immediately and institute safety measures.
2. Remove potentially harmful objects from the patient's immediate environment.
3. If the patient is at high risk for suicide, observe constantly, even when the patient is in bed or using the bathroom.
4. Observe carefully when the patient is taking medication. Check the patient's mouth to ensure that pills have been swallowed. Give medication in liquid form if possible.
5. Explain all safety measures to the patient. Communicate caring and concern.
6. Be particularly wary if the patient suddenly becomes calmer and seems at peace. A suicide plan may have been finalized, resulting in relief of anxiety.

IMPLEMENTATION

Intervening in Self-Destructive Behavior

The highest-priority nursing interventions are those that protect the patient from immediate danger. In addition, the patient requires assistance in increasing self-esteem and in regulating emotions and behaviors. The involvement of family and community support systems is recommended. A **Nursing Treatment Plan Summary for patients with maladaptive self-protective responses** is presented on this page and pages 248-249.

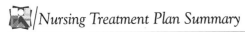

Nursing Treatment Plan Summary

Maladaptive Self-Protective Responses

Nursing Diagnosis: Potential for self-directed violence

Expected Outcome: Patient will not inflict physical self-injury.

Short-Term Goals	Interventions	Rationale
Patient will not engage in self-injury activities.	Observe closely. Remove harmful objects. Provide a safe environment. Provide for basic physiological needs. Contract for safety if appropriate. Monitor medications.	Highest priority is given to lifesaving patient care activities. Patient's behavior must be supervised until self-control is adequate for safety.

Continued

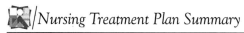

Nursing Treatment Plan Summary

Maladaptive Self-Protective Responses—cont'd

Short-Term Goals	Interventions	Rationale
Patient will identify positive aspects of self.	Identify patient's strengths. Encourage patient to participate in activities that patient likes and does well. Encourage good hygiene and grooming. Foster healthy interpersonal relationships.	Self-destructive behavior reflects underlying depression related to low self-esteem and anger directed inward.
Patient will implement two adaptive self-protective responses.	Facilitate awareness, labeling, and expression of feelings. Assist patient to recognize unhealthy coping mechanisms. Identify alternative means of coping. Reward healthy coping behaviors.	Maladaptive coping mechanisms must be replaced with healthy ones to manage stress and anxiety.
Patient will identify two social support resources that can be helpful.	Assist significant others to communicate constructively with patient. Promote healthy family relationships. Identify relevant community resources. Initiate referrals to community resources.	Social isolation leads to low self-esteem and depression, perpetuating self-destructive behavior.

/*Nursing Treatment Plan Summary*

Maladaptive Self-Protective Responses—cont'd

Short-Term Goals	Interventions	Rationale
Patient will be able to describe the treatment plan and its rationale.	Involve patient and significant others in care planning. Explain characteristics of identified health care needs, nursing care needs, medical diagnosis, and recommended treatment and medications. Elicit response to nursing care plan. Modify plan based on patient feedback.	Understanding of and participation in health care planning enhance compliance.

EVALUATION

1. Have threats to the patient's physical integrity or self-system been reduced in nature, number, origin, or timing?
2. Do the patient's behaviors reflect concern for his or her own physical, psychological, and social well-being?
3. Have the patient's coping resources been adequately assessed and mobilized?
4. Does the patient describe self and behavior accurately and objectively?
5. Is the patient using adaptive coping responses?

6. Does the patient engage in self-enhancing activities?
7. Is the patient taking reasonable risks that promote personal growth?

🔎 Your Internet Connection

American Association of Suicidology
www.suicidology.org

American Foundation for Suicide Prevention
www.afsp.org

National Strategy for Suicide Prevention
www.mentalhealth.org/suicideprevention

Suicide Awareness/Voices of Education (SAVE)
www.save.org

Suicide Prevention Resource Center
www.sprc.org

Surgeon General's Call to Action to Prevent Suicide
www.surgeongeneral.gov/library/calltoaction

■ NEUROBIOLOGICAL RESPONSES

Psychosis refers to the mental state of experiencing reality differently from others. During an episode of psychosis, the patient does not realize others are not experiencing the same things and wonders why others are not reacting in a similar manner. The overall goal of nursing care is to help the patient recognize the psychosis and develop strategies to manage the symptoms.

It is important to remember that these are complex neurobiological brain diseases affecting one's ability to perceive and process information and involving a number of syndromes. The symptoms of psychosis are clustered within five major categories of brain function: (1) cognition, (2) perception, (3) emotion, (4) behavior, and (5) socialization (also referred to as relational).

ASSESSMENT

Behaviors

Schizophrenia is a serious, persistent brain disease that results in psychotic behavior, concrete thinking, and difficulties in information processing, interpersonal relationships, and problem solving. Box 15-1 presents information on how schizophrenia affects the individual and society.

BOX **15-1**

Impact of Schizophrenia on the Individual and Society

- Approximately 1 in every 100 people in the United States (2.5 million) has schizophrenia, regardless of race, ethnic group, or gender.
- In three of four patients, schizophrenia begins between ages 17 and 25.
- Ninety-five percent of patients with schizophrenia have it for their lifetime.
- The cost of family caregiving and crime-related and welfare-related expenditures resulting from schizophrenia is $33 billion annually in the United States.
- More than 75% of taxpayer dollars spent on treatment of mental illness is used for patients with schizophrenia.
- Patients with schizophrenia occupy 25% of all inpatient hospital beds.
- An estimated one third to one half of homeless people in the United States have schizophrenia.
- Schizophrenia is ranked fourth in the top ten diseases worldwide in terms of burden of illness. The top three are unipolar depression, alcohol abuse, and bipolar disorder.
- Schizophrenia is a chronic illness, five times more common than multiple sclerosis, six times more common than insulin-dependent diabetes, 60 times more common than muscular dystrophy, and 80 times more common than Huntington's disease.
- Of patients with schizophrenia, 25% do not respond adequately to traditional antipsychotic medication.
- Approximately 20% to 50% of patients with schizophrenia attempt suicide; 10% succeed.

Related to Cognition. Behaviors related to problems in information processing associated with schizophrenia are often referred to as *cognitive deficits*. They include problems with all aspects of memory, attention, form and content of speech, decision making, and thought content (Box 15-2). Table 15-1 summarizes behaviors related to these problems.

BOX **15-2**

Problems in Cognitive Functioning

Memory

Difficulty retrieving and using stored memory
Impaired short-term/long-term memory

Attention

Difficulty maintaining attention
Poor concentration
Distractibility
Inability to use selective attention

Form and Content of Speech (Formal Thought Disorder)

Loose associations
Tangential/illogical content
Incoherence/word salad/neologism
Circumstantial approach
Pressured/distractible speech
Paucity of speech

Decision Making

Failure to abstract
Indecisiveness
Lack of insight

Continued

BOX 15-2

Problems in Cognitive Functioning—cont'd

Decision Making—cont'd
Impaired concept formation
Impaired judgment
Illogical thinking
Lack of planning and problem-solving skills
Difficulty initiating tasks

Thought Content
Delusions:
  Paranoid
  Grandiose
  Religious
  Somatic
  Nihilistic
  Thought broadcasting
  Thought insertion
  Thought control

Related to Perception. *Perception* refers to identification and initial interpretation of a stimulus based on information received through the five senses. Box 15-3 summarizes behaviors related to problems with perception. Table 15-2 presents sensory modalities involved in hallucinations.

Related to Emotion. Emotions can be *hyperexpressed* or *hypoexpressed* in an incongruent manner. Individuals with schizophrenia typically have problems related to hypoexpression (Box 15-4). These patients also often experience emotions related to the difficulties caused by their illness, such as frustration over barriers to accomplishment of personal goals.

Table 15-1	Behavior Related to Cognitive Problems in Schizophrenia
COGNITIVE PROBLEM	**BEHAVIORS**
Memory	Forgetfulness
	Disinterest
	Lack of compliance
Attention	Difficulty completing tasks
	Difficulty concentrating on work
Form and content of speech	Difficulty communicating thoughts and feelings
Decision making	Difficulty initiating and completing activities
	Concrete thought:
	Inability to carry out multistage commands
	Problems with time management
	Difficulty managing money
	Literal interpretation of words and symbols
Thought content	Delusions

BOX 15-3

Behaviors Related to Perceptual Problems Associated with Maladaptive Neurobiological Responses

Hallucinations
Illusions
Sensory integration problems
Poor visceral pain recognition
Problems with stereognosis (recognition of objects by touch)
Problems with graphesthesia (recognition of letters "drawn" on the skin)
Misidentification of faces (including self)

Table 15-2	Sensory Modalities Involved in Hallucinations
SENSE	CHARACTERISTICS
Auditory	Hearing noises or sounds, usually in the form of voices. Sounds may range from a simple noise or voice, to a voice talking about the patient, to complete conversations between two or more people about the hallucinating patient. Additional types include audible thoughts, in which the patient hears voices that are speaking what the patient is thinking, and commands that tell the patient to do something, sometimes harmful or dangerous.
Visual	Visual stimuli in the form of flashes of light, geometric figures, cartoon figures, and elaborate and complex scenes or visions. Visions can be pleasant or terrifying (e.g., seeing monsters).
Olfactory	Putrid, foul, and rancid smells of a repulsive nature, such as blood, urine, or feces. Occasionally the odors can be pleasant. Olfactory hallucinations are typically associated with stroke, tumor, seizures, and the dementias.
Gustatory	Putrid, foul, and rancid tastes of a repulsive nature, such as blood, urine, or feces.
Tactile	Experiencing pain or discomfort with no apparent stimuli. Feeling electrical sensations coming from the ground, inanimate objects, or other people.
Cenesthetic	Feeling body functions, such as blood pulsing through veins and arteries, food digesting, or urine forming.
Kinesthetic	Sensation of movement while standing motionless.

BOX **15-4**

Emotional Responses Occurring in Schizophrenia

Alexithymia—difficulty naming and describing emotions
Apathy—lack of feelings, emotions, interests, or concern
Anhedonia—inability or decreased ability to experience
   pleasure, joy, intimacy, and closeness

Related to Movement and Behavior. Maladaptive
neurobiological responses cause behaviors that are odd,
unsightly, confusing, difficult to manage, and puzzling to
others (Box 15-5).

BOX **15-5**

Abnormal Movements and Behaviors in
Schizophrenia

Movements
Catatonia, waxy flexibility, posturing
Extrapyramidal side effects of psychotropic medications
Abnormal eye movements
Grimacing
Apraxia (difficulty carrying out a complex task)
Echopraxia (purposeless imitation of others' movements)
Abnormal gait
Mannerisms

Behaviors
Deterioration in appearance
Aggression/agitation
Repetitive or stereotyped behavior
Avolition (lack of energy and drive)
Lack of persistence at work or school

Associated with Socialization. *Socialization* is the ability to form cooperative and interdependent relationships with others. Box 15-6 summarizes behaviors associated with the relational consequences of maladaptive neurobiological responses.

Positive and Negative Symptoms. Finally, the symptoms or behaviors related to schizophrenia have been grouped or categorized in various ways. One prominent system groups them into **positive symptoms** (additional behaviors) and **negative symptoms** (deficit of behaviors). Figure 15-1 presents five core symptom clusters that reflect the full impact this illness can have on the individual and society.

Predisposing Factors

Biological. Various neurodevelopmental abnormalities associated with maladaptive neurobiological responses are only beginning to be understood, as indicated by the following studies:

1. Brain imaging studies have begun to reveal widespread involvement of the brain in the development of schizophrenia. *Lesions* in the frontal, temporal, and limbic areas are related to psychotic behaviors. *Enlarged*

BOX **15-6**

Behaviors Associated with Socialization Resulting from Maladaptive Neurobiological Responses

Social withdrawal and isolation
Low self-esteem
Social inappropriateness
Disinterest in recreational activities
Gender identity confusion
Stigma-related withdrawal by others
Decreased quality of life

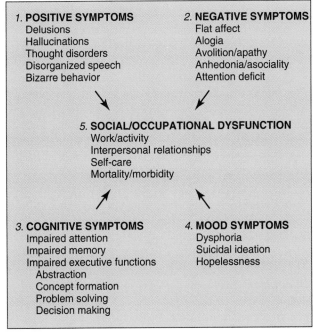

1. **POSITIVE SYMPTOMS**
   Delusions
   Hallucinations
   Thought disorders
   Disorganized speech
   Bizarre behavior

2. **NEGATIVE SYMPTOMS**
   Flat affect
   Alogia
   Avolition/apathy
   Anhedonia/asociality
   Attention deficit

5. **SOCIAL/OCCUPATIONAL DYSFUNCTION**
   Work/activity
   Interpersonal relationships
   Self-care
   Mortality/morbidity

3. **COGNITIVE SYMPTOMS**
   Impaired attention
   Impaired memory
   Impaired executive functions
       Abstraction
       Concept formation
       Problem solving
       Decision making

4. **MOOD SYMPTOMS**
   Dysphoria
   Suicidal ideation
   Hopelessness

Figure 15-1 Core symptom clusters in schizophrenia.

ventricles and *decreased cortical mass* indicate brain atrophy.

2. Several brain chemicals have been implicated in schizophrenia. Research points most strongly to the following:
   - An excess of the neurotransmitter dopamine
   - An imbalance between dopamine and other neurotransmitters, especially serotonin
   - Problems in the dopamine receptor systems

3. Family studies involving twins and adopted children have suggested a *genetic role* for schizophrenia. Identical twins, even when raised separately, have a higher co-occurrence of schizophrenia than nonidentical pairs of

siblings. Recent genetic research focuses on gene mapping in families with a higher incidence of schizophrenia in first-degree relatives compared with the general population.

Psychological. Psychodynamic theories for the development of maladaptive neurobiological responses have not been supported by research. Unfortunately, earlier psychological theories led to families being blamed for these disorders. This results in families lacking trust in mental health professionals.

Sociocultural. Accumulated stress may contribute to the onset of schizophrenia and other psychotic disorders but is not believed to be the primary cause.

Precipitating Stressors

Biological. Biological stressors related to maladaptive neurobiological responses include (1) interference in the brain's communication and feedback loop, which regulate information processing; and (2) abnormal gating (nerve communication involving electrolytes) mechanisms in the brain, resulting in inability to attend to stimuli selectively.

Environmental. A biologically determined threshold for stress tolerance interacts with environmental stressors to determine the occurrence of disturbed behavior.

Symptom Triggers and Stress. Triggers are precursors, stimuli or stressors that often precede a new episode of illness. Box 15-7 lists common triggers of maladaptive neurobiological responses related to the individual's health, environment, attitudes, and behaviors.

Studies of relapse and symptom exacerbation provide evidence that stress, the person's appraisal of the stressor, and problems with coping may predict the return of symptoms. The **stress diathesis model** states that schizophrenic symp-

BOX **15-7**

Symptom Triggers of Maladaptive Neurobiological Responses

Health

Poor nutrition
Lack of sleep
Out-of-balance circadian rhythms
Fatigue
Infection
Central nervous system drugs
Lack of exercise
Barriers to accessing health care

Environment

Hostile/critical environment
Housing difficulties (unsatisfactory housing)
Pressure to perform (loss of independent living)
Changes in life events, daily patterns of activity
Interpersonal difficulties, disruptions in interpersonal
    relationships
Social isolation
Lack of social support
Job pressures (poor occupational skills)
Stigmatization
Poverty
Lack of transportation (resources)
Inability to get/keep a job

Attitudes/Behaviors

"Poor me" (low self-concept)
"Hopeless" (lack of self-confidence)
"I'm a failure" (loss of motivation to use skills)
"Lack of control" (demoralization)
Feeling overpowered by symptoms
"No one likes me" (unable to meet spiritual needs)

Continued

BOX 15-7

Symptom Triggers of Maladaptive Neurobiological Responses—cont'd

Attitudes/Behaviors—cont'd
Looks/acts different from others who are of the same age, culture
Poor social skills
Aggressive behavior
Violent behavior
Poor medication management
Poor symptom management

toms develop based on the relationship between the amount of stress a person experiences and an internal stress tolerance threshold. This is an important model because it integrates biological, psychological, and sociocultural factors in explaining the development of schizophrenia.

Coping Mechanisms

Behaviors that represent efforts to protect the patient from the frightening experiences associated with maladaptive neurobiological responses include the following:

- *Regression*, related to information processing problems and efforts to manage anxiety, leaving little energy for activities of daily living
- *Projection*, as an effort to explain confusing perceptions
- *Withdrawal*

NURSING DIAGNOSIS

The box on page 263 presents the primary and related NANDA nursing diagnoses for maladaptive neurobiological responses. A complete nursing assessment would include all maladaptive responses, and many additional nursing problems would be identified.

NANDA NURSING DIAGNOSES

Related to Maladaptive Neurobiological Responses

Anxiety
Body image, Disturbed
Communication, Impaired verbal*
Confusion, Acute
Coping, Compromised family
Coping, Ineffective
Decisional conflict
Hopelessness
Memory, Impaired
Noncompliance
Personal identity, Disturbed
Role performance, Ineffective
Sedentary lifestyle
Self-care deficit (bathing/hygiene, dressing/grooming)
Sensory perception, Disturbed*
Social interaction, Impaired*
Social isolation
Suicide, Risk for
Therapeutic regimen management, Ineffective
Thought processes, Disturbed*

From North American Nursing Diagnosis Association: NANDA nursing diagnoses: definitions and classification 2005-2006, *Philadelphia, 2005, The Association.*
*Primary nursing diagnosis for maladaptive neurobiological responses.

Related Medical Diagnoses

Maladaptive neurobiological responses are included in the medical diagnostic category of schizophrenia and psychotic disorders. The box on pages 264-266 describes these disorders.

DSM-IV-TR MEDICAL DIAGNOSES

Related to Maladaptive Neurobiological Responses

DSM-IV-TR Diagnosis	Essential Features
Schizophrenia	At least two of the following, each present for a significant time during a 1-month period: 1. Delusions 2. Hallucinations 3. Disorganized speech 4. Grossly disorganized or catatonic behavior 5. Negative symptoms (i.e., flat affect, alogia, avolition) For a significant time since the onset of the disturbance, one or more major areas of functioning (e.g., work, interpersonal relations, self-care) are greatly below the level achieved before the onset.
Paranoid type	Continuous signs of the disturbance persist for at least 6 months.
Disorganized type	Preoccupation with one or more delusions or frequent auditory hallucinations. All the following are prominent: disorganized speech, disorganized behavior, and flat or inappropriate affect; also, does not meet the criteria for catatonic type.
Catatonic type	At least two of the following dominate the clinical picture: motor immobility, as evidenced by catalepsy or stupor; excessive motor activity; extreme negativism or mutism; peculiarities of voluntary movement, as evidenced by posturing, stereotyped movements, prominent mannerisms, or prominent grimacing; echolalia; and echopraxia.
Undifferentiated type	Symptoms meeting the first general criterion for schizophrenia are present, but criteria for other types are not met.

DSM-IV-TR MEDICAL DIAGNOSES

Related to Maladaptive Neurobiological Responses—cont'd

DSM-IV-TR Diagnosis	*Essential Features*
Residual type	Criteria for schizophrenia or any subtype are not met. Continuing evidence of the disturbance is indicated by negative symptoms or attenuated presence of two or more symptoms included in the general criteria.
Schizophreniform disorder	Meets criteria for schizophrenia, and an episode lasts at least 1 month but less than 6 months. "With" or "without" good prognostic features is specified based on at least two of the following: onset of prominent psychotic symptoms within 4 weeks of first noticeable change in behavior or functioning; confusion or perplexity at the height of the psychosis; good premorbid social and occupational functioning; and absence of blunted or flat affect.
Schizoaffective disorder	Interrupted period of illness, including a major depressive episode or manic episode, concurrent with symptoms of schizophrenia. During the same period of illness, delusions or hallucinations have occurred for at least 2 weeks in the absence of prominent mood symptoms. Symptoms of a mood episode are present during a substantial part of the illness. The condition is not caused by substance abuse or a general medical illness.
Delusional disorder	Nonbizarre delusions (i.e., situations that could occur, such as being followed, being poisoned, or having a disease) lasting at least a month. Has never met criteria for schizophrenia. Apart from the impact of the delusion, functioning and behavior are not greatly affected.

Continued

DSM-IV-TR MEDICAL DIAGNOSES

Related to Maladaptive Neurobiological Responses—cont'd

DSM-IV-TR Diagnosis	Essential Features
Brief psychotic disorder	Presence of at least one of the following: delusions, hallucinations, disorganized speech, and grossly disorganized or catatonic behavior (behaviors are not culturally sanctioned). Duration of 1 day to 1 month, with eventual return to premorbid functioning. Presence (brief reactive psychosis) or absence of marked stressors.
Shared psychotic disorder (folie à deux)	A delusion develops in an individual in the context of a close relationship with someone who already has a delusion. The delusions of those involved are similar in content.

Modified from American Psychiatric Association: Diagnostic and statistical manual of mental disorders, *ed 4, Text Revision (DSM-IV-TR), Washington, DC, 2000, The Association.*

OUTCOME IDENTIFICATION

The expected outcome when working with a patient with maladaptive neurobiological responses is:

The patient will live, learn, and work at the maximal level of success possible, as defined by the individual.

PLANNING

A **Family Education Plan for understanding psychosis** is presented on pages 267-269.

FAMILY EDUCATION PLAN

UNDERSTANDING PSYCHOSIS

Content	Instructional Activities	Evaluation
Describe psychosis	Introduce participants and leaders. State purpose of group. Define terminology associated with psychosis.	Participant describes the characteristics of psychosis.
Identify the causes of psychotic disorders.	Present theories of psychotic disorders. Use audiovisual aids to explain brain anatomy, brain biochemistry, and major neurotransmitters.	Participant discusses the relationship between brain anatomy, brain biochemistry, and major neurotransmitters and the development of psychosis.
Define schizophrenia according to symptoms and diagnostic criteria.	Lead a discussion of the diagnostic criteria for schizophrenia. Show a film on schizophrenia.	Participant describes the symptoms and diagnostic criteria for schizophrenia.
Describe the relationship between anxiety and psychotic disorders.	Present types and stages of anxiety. Discuss steps in reducing and resolving anxiety.	Participant identifies and describes the stages of anxiety and ways to reduce or resolve it.

Continued

FAMILY EDUCATION PLAN

UNDERSTANDING PSYCHOSIS—CONT'D

Content	Instructional Activities	Evaluation
Analyze the impact of living with hallucinations.	Describe the characteristics of hallucinations. Demonstrate ways to communicate with someone who is hallucinating.	Participant demonstrates effective ways to communicate with a person who has hallucinations.
Analyze the impact of living with delusions.	Describe types of delusions. Demonstrate ways to communicate with someone who has delusions. Discuss interventions for delusions.	Participant demonstrates effective ways to communicate with a person who has delusions.
Discuss the use of psychotropic medications and the role of nutrition.	Provide and explain handouts describing the characteristics of psychotropic medications prescribed for schizophrenia.	Participant identifies and describes the characteristics of medications prescribed for self or family member.
Describe the characteristics of relapse and the role of compliance with the therapeutic regimen.	Assist participants to describe their own experiences with relapse. Discuss symptom management techniques and the importance of complying with the therapeutic regimen.	Participant describes behaviors that indicate an impending relapse and discusses the importance of symptom management and compliance with the therapeutic regimen.

Family Education Plan

Understanding Psychosis—cont'd

Content	Instructional Activities	Evaluation
Analyze behaviors that promote wellness.	Discuss the components of wellness. Relate wellness to the elements of symptom management.	Participant analyzes the effect of maintaining a state of wellness on the occurrence of symptoms.
Discuss ways to cope adaptively while living with psychosis.	Lead a group discussion focused on the daily problems of living with psychosis and on coping behaviors. Propose ways to create a low-stress environment.	Participant describes ways to modify lifestyle to create a low-stress environment.

IMPLEMENTATION

Empirically validated treatments related to schizophrenia are summarized in Table 15-3.

Nursing interventions may include a broad range of psychosocial and psychobiological treatments and are based on the nurse's assessment of the patient's needs and strengths. Significant others are included whenever possible. The major approaches for nursing intervention with patients who have maladaptive neurobiological responses are summarized as follows:

1. **Behavioral strategies.** Table 15-4 presents strategies for nurses working with patients who have psychoses.

Table 15-3	Summarizing the Evidence on Neurobiological Responses
DISORDER	**TREATMENT**
Schizophrenia	• Behavioral therapy and social-learning-token-economy programs help structure, support, and reinforce prosocial behavior in persons with schizophrenia.
	• Structured, educational family interventions help patients with schizophrenia maintain gains achieved with medication and case management.
	• Social skills training has enabled persons with schizophrenia to acquire instrumental and affiliative skills to improve functioning in their communities.
	• Pharmacological treatment has had a profoundly positive impact on the course of schizophrenia. The introduction of atypical antipsychotics is promising because of their reduced side effects and enhanced efficacy in some patients.

From Nathan P, Gorman J: *A guide to treatments that work*, ed 2, New York, 2002, Oxford University Press.

2. **Managing delusions.** Box 15-8 presents strategies for working with delusional patients, and Box 15-9 lists barriers to intervention for delusions.
3. **Managing hallucinations.** Box 15-10 outlines strategies for working with patients to help them cope with ongoing hallucinations.
4. **Psychopharmacology.** Antipsychotic medications are described in Chapter 21.

Text continued on page 280.

Table 15-4	Behavioral Strategies for Patients With Psychosis
CORE PROBLEM	**NURSING INTERVENTIONS**
Difficulty assessing passage of time	Teach patient how to use clocks to tell time. Teach patient to use environmental cues (e.g., sun going down, certain radio program) to orient self to time of day. Assist patient in creating and maintaining a calendar of scheduled activities.
Concrete thinking	Realize patient sees every problem as having one solution. Teach patient to consider other possible solutions to problems. Realize patient frequently thinks there is only one way to do a task. Create alternative methods to approach situations.
Difficulty telling background from foreground information	Teach patient to distinguish between important and unimportant information. Teach patient to focus on only the important information. Help patient learn to avoid or minimize confusion caused by excess stimulation from noise, large crowds, etc.
Slowed information processing	Give patient time to process and respond to information. Minimize anxiety, which increases information processing difficulties. Demonstrate genuine interest in trying to understand what patient is saying. Use clear and simple language when communicating with patient.

Continued

Table 15-4	Behavioral Strategies for Patients With Psychosis—cont'd
CORE PROBLEM	**NURSING INTERVENTIONS**
Difficulty screening information to share	Teach patient to identify people who patient can talk to about the illness. Teach patient to contact these people when the symptoms are creating problems. Let patient know you understand the illness and are a "safe person" to talk with.
Communication difficulties	Use active listening to understand patient. Clarify what patient is trying to convey. Listen for the theme. Seek validation from patient on what is communicated. Help patient with vocabulary as needed. Use the literal meaning of words. Have patient repeat what was heard. Help patient understand the words and phrases used.
Problems expressing needs	Assist patient to identify and prioritize needs. Assist patient to express needs in ways that others will understand. Role-play conversations and practice negotiating with others.
Low self-concept	Help patient identify and maximize strengths and positive characteristics. Use role play to handle common situations that patients face. Give positive feedback when patient handles a situation well. Help problem-solve a negative situation to determine how it could have been better handled.

Table 15-4	Behavioral Strategies for Patients With Psychosis—cont'd
CORE PROBLEM	**NURSING INTERVENTIONS**
Forced isolation resulting from stigma	Maximize patient's understanding of the illness.
	Teach patient to minimize stigmatizing behaviors when possible.
	Identify comments that are difficult for patient to confront.
	Teach ways to handle stigma and rude comments.
	Develop concrete humorous comebacks.
	Role-play various situations with nurse being the patient.
Difficulty with perception and interpretation of sensory stimuli	Review problematic situations with patient.
	List and assess the thought processes in interpreting events.
	Help patient reality-test and reframe problematic interpretations.
	Reinforce positive and productive processes.
Poor attention span and difficulty completing tasks	Help patient break tasks into small, sequential steps.
	Help patient keep focused on a single task, a step at a time.
	Do not emphasize completing the task.
	Give directions to patient one step at a time.
Inappropriate social behaviors	Identify patient's thought processes that lead to the behavior.
	Ask patient about the behavior.
	Help correct inaccurate perceptions.
	Help patient identify undesirable outcomes of the behavior.
	Teach appropriate social skills.

Continued

Table 15-4	Behavioral Strategies for Patients With Psychosis—cont'd
CORE PROBLEM	**NURSING INTERVENTIONS**
Difficulty with decision making	Assist patient to decide on desired outcomes.
	Help patient prioritize goals and categorize them into short term and long term.
	Help patient establish a timeline for attainment of each goal.
	Help patient establish small, concrete steps to achieve desired goals.
	Ensure these small steps are achievable by patient and are congruent with patient's culture and values.

BOX 15-8

Strategies for Working With Patients With Delusions

Place the delusion in a time frame and identify triggers.

- Identify all the components of the delusion by placing it in time and sequence.
- Identify triggers that may be related to stress or anxiety.
- If delusions are linked to anxiety, teach anxiety management skills.
- Develop a symptom management program.

Assess the intensity, frequency, and duration of the delusion.

- Help the patient dispel fleeting delusions in a short time frame.
- Consider temporarily avoiding fixed delusions, or those endured over time, to prevent them from becoming stumbling blocks in the nurse-patient relationship.
- Listen quietly until there is no need to discuss the delusion.

BOX **15-8**

Strategies for Working With Patients With Delusions—cont'd

Identify emotional components of the delusion.
- Respond to the patient's underlying feelings rather than the illogical nature of the delusions.
- Encourage discussion of the patient's fears, anxiety, and anger without assuming the delusion is right or wrong.

Observe for evidence of concrete thinking.
- Determine whether or not the patient takes you literally.
- Determine if you and the patient are using language in the same way.

Observe speech for symptoms of a thought disorder.
- Determine if the patient exhibits a thought disorder (e.g., talking in circles, going off on tangents, easily changing subjects, unable to respond to your attempts to redirect).
- Realize that it may not be the appropriate time to point out discrepancies between fact and delusion.

Observe for the ability to use cause-and-effect reasoning accurately.
- Determine if the patient can make logical predictions (inductive or deductive) based on past experiences.
- Determine if the patient can conceptualize time.
- Determine if the patient can access and use recent and long-term memory meaningfully.

Continued

BOX **15-8**

Strategies for Working With Patients With Delusions—cont'd

Distinguish between description of the experience and facts of the situation.

- Identify false beliefs about real situations.
- Promote the patient's ability to reality-test.
- Determine if the patient is hallucinating, because this will strengthen the delusion.

Carefully question the facts as they are presented and their meaning.

- Talk about the delusion to try to help the patient see it is not true.
- Note that if this step is taken before the previous steps are completed, it may reinforce the delusion.

Discuss the delusion and its consequences.

- When intensity of the delusion lessens, discuss the delusion when the patient is ready.
- Discuss the consequences of the delusion.
- Allow the patient to take responsibility for behavior, daily activities, and decision making.
- Encourage the patient's personal responsibility for and participation in wellness and recovery.

Promote distraction as a way to stop focusing on the delusion.

- Promote activities that require attention to physical skills and that will help the patient use time constructively.
- Recognize and reinforce healthy and positive aspects of the patient's personality.

BOX **15-9**

Barriers to Successful Intervention for Delusions

Becoming anxious and avoiding the patient

This leads to annoyance, anger, a sense of hopelessness and failure, feelings of inadequacy, and potential laughing at or discounting of the patient.

Reinforcing the delusion

Do not agree with the delusion, especially to obtain the patient's cooperation.

Attempting to prove the patient is wrong

Do not attempt a logical explanation.

Setting unrealistic goals

Do not underestimate the power of a delusion and the patient's need for it.

Becoming incorporated into the delusional system

This will cause great confusion for the patient and make it impossible to establish the boundaries of the therapeutic relationship.

Failing to clarify confusion surrounding the delusion

If the nurse does not clearly understand the complexity and many intricacies of the delusion, the delusion will become more elaborate.

Being inconsistent in intervention

The nurse must firmly adhere to the intervention plan. "Try anything" approaches lead to inconsistency, and the patient is less able to identify reality.

Seeing the delusion first and the patient second

Avoid using such phrases as, "The person who thinks he's being poisoned."

BOX **15-10**

**Strategies for Working With Patients
With Hallucinations**

Establish a trusting, interpersonal relationship.

- Remember that if you are anxious or frightened, the patient will be anxious or frightened.
- Be patient, show acceptance, and use active listening skills.

Assess for symptoms of hallucinations, including duration, intensity, and frequency.

- Observe for behavioral clues that indicate the presence of hallucinations.
- Observe for clues that identify the level of intensity and duration of the hallucination.
- Help the patient record the number of hallucinations experienced each day.

Focus on symptoms and ask patient to describe what is happening.

- Empower the patient by helping to understand the symptoms experienced or demonstrated.
- Help the patient gain control of the hallucinations, seek helpful distractions, and minimize intensity.

Explore drug and alcohol use.

- Determine if the patient is using alcohol or drugs (over-the-counter, prescription, or street drugs).
- Determine if these may be responsible for or may exacerbate the hallucinations.

BOX **15-10**

Strategies for Working With Patients With Hallucinations—cont'd

If the patient asks, simply say you are not experiencing the same stimuli.

- Respond by letting the patient know what is actually happening in the environment.
- Do not argue with the patient about differences in perceptions.
- When a hallucination occurs, do not leave the patient alone.

Suggest and reinforce the use of interpersonal relationships as a symptom management technique.

- Encourage the patient to talk to someone trusted who will give supportive and corrective feedback.
- Assist the patient in mobilizing social supports.

Help the patient describe and compare current and past hallucinations.

- Determine if there is a pattern to the patient's hallucinations.
- Encourage the patient to remember when hallucinations first began.
- Pay attention to the content of the hallucination because it may provide clues for predicting behavior.
- Be especially alert for "command" hallucinations that may "compel" the patient to act in a certain way.
- Encourage the patient to describe past and present thoughts, feelings, and actions as they relate to hallucinations.

Continued

BOX 15-10

**Strategies for Working With Patients
With Hallucinations—cont'd**

**Help the patient identify needs that may be
reflected in the content of the hallucination.**
- Identify needs that may trigger hallucinations.
- Focus on the patient's unmet needs, and discuss their
  relationship to the presence of hallucinations.

**Determine the impact of the patient's symptoms
on activities of daily living.**
- Provide feedback regarding the patient's general coping
  responses and activities of daily living.
- Help the patient recognize symptoms, symptom
  triggers, and symptom management strategies.

5. **Managing relapse.** Patients and their family members
   should be informed about how to identify and take
   action when a relapse is impending. Box 15-11 lists
   nursing interventions directed toward preventing

BOX 15-11

Nursing Interventions to Prevent Relapse

- Identify symptoms that signal relapse.
- Identify symptom triggers.
- Select symptom management techniques.
- Identify coping strategies for symptom triggers.
- Identify support system for future relapse.
- Document action plan in written form and file with key
  support people.
- Facilitate patient's integration into family and
  community.

relapse, and Box 15-12 is a patient guide for potential relapse.

6. **Patient and family education.** Patients and their families are much better able to manage the illness if they are provided with information about diagnosis, medications, current research, and community resources.

BOX **15-12**

Patient Guide for Handling Potential Relapse

1. **Go to a safe environment** with someone who can assist you if help is needed. This person should be able to monitor behavior that indicates the relapse is becoming worse.
2. **Reduce the stress and demands on you.** This includes reducing stimuli. Some people find a quiet room where they can be alone, perhaps with soft music. Consider using relaxation or distraction techniques. A quiet place where you can talk with a person you trust is often helpful.
3. **Take medications** if this is part of your program. Work with your prescriber to determine if medications may be useful to reduce relapse. Medications are most helpful when used in a safe, quiet environment and with stress reduction techniques.
4. **Talk to a trusted person** about what the voices are saying to you or about the thoughts you are having. The person needs to know ahead of time that you will call if you need help.
5. **Avoid negative people** who make such comments as, "You're thinking crazy" or "Stop that negative talk."
6. **Patient and family education.** Patients and their families are much better able to manage the illness if they are provided with information about diagnosis, medications, current research, and community resources.

A **Nursing Treatment Plan Summary** for the patient with maladaptive neurobiological responses is presented below and on pages 283-286.

/*Nursing Treatment Plan Summary*

Maladaptive Neurobiological Responses

Nursing Diagnosis: Altered thought processes

Expected Outcome: Patient will live, learn, and work at the maximal level of success possible, as defined by the individual.

Short-Term Goals	Interventions	Rationale
Patient will participate in brief, regularly scheduled meetings with nurse.	Initiate a nurse-patient relationship contract mutually agreed on by nurse and patient. Schedule brief (5- to 10-minute) frequent contacts with patient. Consistently approach patient at scheduled time. Extend length of sessions gradually based on patient's agreement.	Establishment of a trusting relationship is fundamental to developing open communication. A patient with altered thought processes cannot tolerate extended, intrusive interactions and functions best in a structured environment.

/*Nursing Treatment Plan Summary*

Maladaptive Neurobiological Responses—cont'd

Short-Term Goals	Interventions	Rationale
Patient will describe delusions and other altered thought processes.	Demonstrate attitude of caring and concern. Validate the meaning of communications with patient. Assist patient to identify the difference between reality and internal thought processes.	Patients are very sensitive to others' responses to their symptoms. A respectful, interested approach enables patient to discuss unusual and frightening thoughts. Identification of reality by a trusted person is helpful.
Patient will identify and describe the effect of brain disease on thought processes.	Provide information about causes of psychoses. Discuss relationship between patient's behaviors and brain function. Involve significant others in educational sessions.	Understanding physiological basis for altered thought processes assists patient to recognize symptoms and to feel in control of the illness. Significant others can provide support and experience less stigma if they are informed about the illness.

Continued

/Nursing Treatment Plan Summary

Maladaptive Neurobiological Responses—cont'd		
Short-Term Goals	**Interventions**	**Rationale**
Patient will identify the signs of impending relapse and describe actions to take to prevent relapse.	Assist patient and significant others to identify behaviors related to altered thought processes that indicate threatened relapse. Identify community resources, and mutually plan actions directed toward prevention of relapse.	Relapse can be predicted if patient and family are alert to warning signs. Early intervention allows patient to be in control of the course of the illness. Family members can be helpful in assisting patient to identify symptoms and in providing support for seeking assistance.
Patient will describe symptom management techniques that are helpful in living with altered thought processes.	Describe symptom management techniques that other patients have used. Ask patient to describe techniques used to manage symptoms. Encourage patient to take control of the illness by using symptom management techniques.	Many patients with psychoses continue to have delusions after the acute phase of the illness has passed. They can function better if they learn ways to manage the symptoms.

/*Nursing Treatment Plan Summary*

Maladaptive Neurobiological Responses—cont'd

Short-Term Goals	Interventions	Rationale
Nursing Diagnosis: Social isolation		
Expected Outcome: Patient will live, learn, and work at the maximal level of success possible, as defined by the individual.		
Patient will engage in a trusting relationship with nurse.	Initiate a nurse-patient relationship contract mutually agreed on by nurse and patient. Establish mutual goals related to social interaction. Establish trust by consistently meeting the elements of the plan and engaging in open and honest communication.	Patients who have maladaptive neurobiological responses often have difficulty trusting others. Difficulty with information processing causes problems interpreting the communication of others.
Patient will discuss personal goals related to social interaction.	Encourage patient to describe current relationship patterns. Discuss past relationship experiences. Identify problems associated with social interaction. Explore goals.	Patient may be unaware of the characteristics of mutually satisfying interpersonal relationships. Honest feedback from nurse can assist patient to identify the reasons for past problems.

Continued

/*Nursing Treatment Plan Summary*

Maladaptive Neurobiological Responses—cont'd

Short-Term Goals	Interventions	Rationale
		Knowledge of patient's relationship goals leads to development of realistic behavioral change.
Patient will identify behaviors that interfere with social relationships.	Share observations about patient's behavior in social situations.	Identification of problematic behavior helps patient and nurse target changes.
Patient will practice alternative social behaviors with nurse.	Discuss possible behavioral changes that will facilitate establishment of social relationships. Role-play alternative behaviors. Provide feedback.	Practice helps patient feel comfortable with new behaviors. Feedback provides reinforcement for successful behavioral change.

EVALUATION

1. Is the patient able to describe the behaviors that characterize the onset of a relapse?
2. Is the patient able to identify and describe the medications prescribed, the reason for taking them, the frequency of taking them, and the possible side effects?
3. Does the patient participate in relationships with other people at a level that is comfortable for the patient?
4. Is the patient's family aware of the characteristics of the illness and able to participate in a supportive relationship with the patient?
5. Are the patient and family informed about available community resources, such as rehabilitation programs, mental health care providers, educational programs, and support groups, and do they use them?

 Your Internet Connection

All About Schizophrenia–Mental Help Net
http://mentalhelp.net/poc/center_index.php?id=7

Consultant for Pharmacotherapy of Schizophrenia
www.mhc.com/Algorithms/Schizophrenia/index.htm

NARSAD: National Alliance for Research on Schizophrenia and Depression
www.narsad.org

The Schizophrenia Home Page
www.schizophrenia.com

World Fellowship for Schizophrenia and Allied Disorders
www.world-schizophrenia.org

SOCIAL RESPONSES AND PERSONALITY DISORDERS

■ SOCIAL RESPONSES

Humans are socially oriented. To achieve satisfaction with life, they must establish positive interpersonal relationships. In a healthy interpersonal relationship the individuals involved are close to each other while maintaining separate identities. The persons also must establish interdependence, which is a balance of dependence and independence in the relationship.

Personality disorders are usually recognizable by adolescence or earlier and continue throughout most of adulthood. They are enduring, inflexible, and maladaptive patterns of response that are severe enough to cause either dysfunctional behavior or profound distress.

Personality disorders are relatively common in the United States; an estimated 10% to 18% of the general population have these illnesses. However, only one fifth of these people are receiving treatment. At least some of these disorders are also associated with greater mortality resulting from suicide.

 ASSESSMENT

Behaviors

The behaviors observed in people with personality disorders are characterized by chronic, maladaptive social responses. The DSM-IV-TR has grouped the personality disorders into three clusters based on descriptive similarities. Table 16-1

Table 16-1	Classification and Features of DSM-IV-TR Personality Disorders
DISORDER	**FEATURES**

Cluster A: Odd, Eccentric, General Tendency Toward Social and Emotional Withdrawal

Paranoid	Distrust: persistently suspicious, secretive, withholding, hypervigilant, jealous, envious
Schizoid	Social detachment: self-absorbed; restricted emotionality; cold and indifferent; neither desires nor enjoys close relationships; anhedonic, indifferent to others; less disturbed than schizotypal
Schizotypal	Interpersonal deficits; cognitive distortions; eccentricities; paranoid; difficulty feeling understood and accepted; odd beliefs, magical thinking, unusual perceptual experiences; social isolation

Cluster B: Overemotional, Dramatic, Erratic, Impulsive

Antisocial	Disregard for the rights of others; lies; manipulates; exploitative; seductive; repeatedly performs acts that are grounds for arrest
Borderline	Instability; impulsivity; hypersensitivity; self-destructive behavior; profound mood shifts; unstable and intense interpersonal relationships
Histrionic	Excessive emotionality; attention seeking; superficial and stormy relationships; lively; uncomfortable when not the center of attention
Narcissistic	Arrogance; need for admiration; lack of empathy; seductive; socially exploitative; manipulative; grandiose sense of self-importance

Continued

Table 16-1	Classification and Features of DSM-IV-TR Personality Disorders—cont'd
DISORDER	FEATURES
Cluster C: Anxious, Fearful	
Avoidant	Social inhibition; withdraw from social and occupational situations that involve significant interpersonal contact; longs for relationships; inadequacy; hypersensitivity to negative criticism, rejection, or shame
Dependent	Submissive behavior; low self-esteem; dependency in relationships; extreme self-consciousness; urgently and indiscriminately seeks another relationship when close relationship ends; inadequate; helpless
Obsessive-compulsive	Unable to express affection; overly cold and rigid; crippling preoccupation with trivial detail, orderliness, perfectionism, and control (i.e., attends to rules, lists, organization, schedules, to the extent that the major point of the activity is lost); superior attitudes

presents a specific classification of interpersonal and behavioral characteristics associated with each of the personality disorders.

People with cluster B personality disorders have unique character features that at times make nursing care complicated and difficult. Frequently occurring maladaptive responses of patients with cluster B personality disorders include manipulation, narcissism, and impulsivity; Table 16-2 lists behaviors related to these responses.

Predisposing Factors

Although much research has been done on disorders that affect interpersonal relationships, no specific conclusions

Table 16-2	Behaviors Related to Maladaptive Social Responses
MALADAPTIVE RESPONSE	BEHAVIORS
Manipulation	Treats others as objects
	Centers relationships around control issues
	Is self-oriented or goal oriented, not oriented to others
Narcissism	Fragile self-esteem
	Constant seeking of praise and admiration
	Egocentric attitude
	Envy
	Rage when others are not supportive
Impulsivity	Inability to plan
	Inability to learn from experience
	Poor judgment
	Unreliability

exist about their causes. A combination of factors is probably involved, including the following:

1. *Developmental factors.* Disrupted family systems may contribute to the development of these responses. Some believe that persons who have these problems were unsuccessful at separating and individuating themselves from their parents. Family norms may discourage relationships outside the family. Family roles are often blurred. Parental alcoholism and child abuse also predispose the person to maladaptive social responses.

2. *Biological factors.* Genetic factors may contribute to maladaptive social responses. Early evidence suggests involvement of the neurotransmitters in the development of these disorders, but further research is needed.

3. *Sociocultural factors.* Social isolation is a major factor in disturbed relationships. This may result from

transience; norms discouraging approaching others; or the devaluing of less productive members of society, such as elderly, disabled, and chronically ill persons. Isolation may result from the adoption of norms, behaviors, and value systems that differ from those of the majority culture. Unrealistic expectations for relationships is another factor related to these disorders.

Precipitating Stressors

Precipitating stressors generally involve stressful life events, such as losses, that interfere with the person's ability to relate to others and cause anxiety. They can be grouped into the following two categories:

1. *Sociocultural stressors.* Stress can arise from decreased stability of the family unit and separation from significant others, such as from hospitalization.
2. *Psychological stressors.* Prolonged or extremely intense anxiety coexists with a limited ability to cope. Demands to separate from significant others or failure of others to meet dependency needs may cause high levels of anxiety.

Coping Mechanisms

Individuals who have maladaptive social responses use a variety of mechanisms in an effort to cope with anxiety. They relate to two specific types of relationship problems as follows:

1. Coping associated with antisocial personality disorder
   Projection
   Splitting
   Devaluation of others
2. Coping associated with borderline personality disorder

Splitting	Idealization of others
Reaction formation	Devaluation of others
Projection	Projective identification
Isolation	

NURSING DIAGNOSIS

Maladaptive social responses may lead to a range of specific disorders at various levels of severity. The nurse must assess the nature of the patient's disorder and consider the range of behaviors presented.

The box below presents the primary and related NANDA nursing diagnoses for maladaptive social responses. A complete nursing assessment would include all maladaptive responses of the patient, and many additional nursing problems would be identified.

NANDA NURSING DIAGNOSES

Related to Maladaptive Social Responses

Anxiety
Coping, Defensive*
Family processes, Interrupted
Role performance, Ineffective
Self-esteem, Chronic low*
Self-mutilation, Risk for*
Social interaction, Impaired*
Violence, Risk for self-directed or other-directed*

From North American Nursing Diagnosis Association: NANDA nursing diagnoses: definitions and classification 2005-2006, Philadelphia, 2005, The Association.
*Primary nursing diagnosis for maladaptive social responses.

Related Medical Diagnoses

Many medically diagnosed psychiatric disorders involve problems with interpersonal relationships. They range in severity from personality disorders to psychoses. The box on pages 294-295 describes these disorders.

DSM-IV-TR MEDICAL DIAGNOSES

Related to Maladaptive Social Responses

DSM-IV-TR Diagnosis	Essential Features
Paranoid personality disorder	Pervasive distrust and suspiciousness of others such that their motives are interpreted as malevolent; beginning in early adulthood and present in a variety of contexts.
Schizoid personality disorder	Pervasive pattern of detachment from social relationships and a restricted range of expression of emotions in interpersonal settings; beginning in early adulthood and present in a variety of contexts.
Schizotypal personality disorder	Pervasive pattern of social and interpersonal deficits marked by acute discomfort with and reduced capacity for close relationships and by cognitive and perceptual distortions and eccentricities of behavior; beginning in early adulthood and present in a variety of contexts.
Antisocial personality disorder	Pervasive pattern of disregard for and violation of the rights of others occurring since age 15.
Borderline personality disorder	Pervasive pattern of instability in interpersonal relationships, self-image, and affect and marked impulsivity; beginning by early adulthood and present in a variety of contexts.
Histrionic personality disorder	Pervasive pattern of excessive emotionality and attention seeking; beginning by early adulthood and present in a variety of contexts.
Narcissistic personality disorder	Pervasive pattern of grandiosity (in fantasy or behavior), need for admiration, and lack of empathy; beginning by early adulthood and present in a variety of contexts.

Modified from American Psychiatric Association: Diagnostic and statistical manual of mental disorders, *ed 4, text revision (DSM-IV-TR), Washington, DC, 2000, The Association.*   *Continued*

DSM-IV-TR MEDICAL DIAGNOSES

Related to Maladaptive Social Responses

DSM-IV-TR Diagnosis	*Essential Features*
Avoidant personality disorder	Pervasive pattern of social inhibition, feelings of inadequacy, and hypersensitivity to negative evaluation; beginning by early adulthood and present in a variety of contexts.
Dependent personality disorder	Pervasive and excessive need to be taken care of that leads to submissive and clinging behaviors and fears of separation; beginning by early adulthood and present in a variety of contexts.
Obsessive-compulsive personality disorder	Pervasive pattern of preoccupation with orderliness, perfectionism, and mental and interpersonal control, at the expense of flexibility, openness, and efficiency; beginning by early adulthood and present in a variety of contexts.

OUTCOME IDENTIFICATION

The expected outcome for a patient with maladaptive social responses is as follows:

The patient will obtain maximal interpersonal satisfaction by establishing and maintaining self-enhancing relationships with others.

PLANNING

A **Patient Education Plan for modifying impulsive behavior** is presented on pages 296-297.

PATIENT EDUCATION PLAN

MODIFYING IMPULSIVE BEHAVIOR

Content	Instructional Activities	Evaluation
Describe characteristics and consequences of impulsive behavior.	Select a situation in which impulsive behavior occurred. Ask patient to describe what happened. Instruct patient to keep a diary of impulsive actions, including a description of events before and after the incident.	Patient identifies and describes an impulsive incident. Patient maintains a diary of impulsive behaviors. Patient explores the causes and consequences of impulsive behavior.
Describe behaviors characteristic of interpersonal anxiety; relate anxiety to impulsive behavior.	Discuss the diary with patient. Assist patient to identify interpersonal anxiety related to impulsive behavior.	Patient connects feelings of interpersonal anxiety with impulsive behavior.
Explain stress reduction techniques.	Describe the stress response. Demonstrate relaxation exercises. Assist patient to return the demonstration.	Patient performs relaxation exercises when signs of anxiety appear.
Identify alternative responses to anxiety-producing situations.	Using situations from the diary and knowledge of relaxation exercises; assist patient to list possible alternative responses.	Patient identifies at least two alternative responses to each anxiety-producing situation.

PATIENT EDUCATION PLAN

MODIFYING IMPULSIVE BEHAVIOR—CONT'D

Content	Instructional Activities	Evaluation
Practice using alternative responses to anxiety-producing situations.	Role-play each of the identified alternative behaviors. Discuss the feelings associated with impulsive behavior and the alternatives.	Patient describes the relationship between behavior and feelings. Patient selects and performs anxiety-reducing behaviors.

IMPLEMENTATION

Empirically validated treatments for some of the medical diagnoses related to personality disorders are summarized in Table 16-3.

The essential elements of nursing intervention with the patient who has maladaptive social responses include the following:

1. Establishing a therapeutic relationship
2. Involving the family to promote and maintain positive change
3. Providing a therapeutic milieu that focuses on realistic expectations, involving the patient in decision making, and processing interactional behaviors in current situations
4. Setting limits and providing structure
5. Protecting the patient from self-harm
6. Focusing on the patient's strengths
7. Implementing contracts and other cognitive-behavioral strategies

Table 16-3	Summarizing the Evidence on Personality Disorders
DISORDER	**TREATMENT**
Avoidant personality disorder	• Group administered behavioral interventions are effective in improving social skills. • Antidepressants may be helpful as well.
Borderline personality disorder	• Dialectical behavioral therapy (DBT) produces lower attrition, fewer and less severe episodes of parasuicidal behavior, and fewer days of hospitalization. • Partial hospitalization involving group and individual psychotherapy for 18 months decreases the number of suicidal attempts, acts of self-harm, psychiatric symptoms, and inpatient days and increases the quality of social and interpersonal functioning. • Noradrenergic agents tend to improve mood but not irritability or dyscontrol. • Serotonergic agents may act to decrease impulsivity.
Mixed personality disorder (excluding cluster A disorders)	• An average of 40 weeks of brief dynamic therapy yields substantial symptomatic improvement at both the end of treatment and after 1.5 years. • Medications may be useful for several of these disorders, although many methodological problems remain to be worked out.
Schizotypal personality disorder (and other cluster A disorders)	• Antipsychotic medications may be useful in reducing some of the symptoms of these disorders.

From Nathan P, Gorman J: *A guide to treatments that work*, ed 2, New York, 2002, Oxford University Press.

A **Nursing Treatment Plan Summary** for the patient who has maladaptive social responses is presented below and on pages 300-303.

/*Nursing Treatment Plan Summary*

Maladaptive Social Responses

Nursing Diagnosis: Impaired social interaction

Expected Outcome: Patient will obtain maximal interpersonal satisfaction by establishing and maintaining self-enhancing relationships with others.

Short-Term Goals	Interventions	Rationale
Patient will participate in a therapeutic nurse-patient relationship.	Initiate a nurse-patient relationship contract mutually agreed on by patient and nurse. Develop mutual behavioral goals. Maintain consistent behavior by all nursing staff. Communicate honest responses to patient's behavior. Provide honest, immediate feedback about behavioral change. Maintain confidentiality. Demonstrate accessibility.	An atmosphere of trust facilitates open expression of thoughts and feelings; a trusting relationship enables patient to risk sharing feelings; honest responses reinforce openness; staff consistency creates a predictable environment that creates trust.

Continued

/*Nursing Treatment Plan Summary*

Maladaptive Social Responses—cont'd

Short-Term Goals	Interventions	Rationale
Patient will describe interpersonal strengths and weaknesses.	Provide patient with opportunities to demonstrate strengths (e.g., helping other patients, assuming leadership roles). Assist patient to analyze experiences perceived as failures. Communicate acceptance of patient as a person while not accepting maladaptive social behavior.	Patient with maladaptive social responses is unable to identify accurately interpersonal strengths and weaknesses, leading to fear of closeness and fear of failure. Nurse must assist patient to separate behavioral incidents from total self-worth and to recognize that patient can be liked even if imperfect.

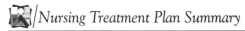

Nursing Treatment Plan Summary

Maladaptive Social Responses—cont'd

Short-Term Goals	Interventions	Rationale
Patient will establish or reestablish one interpersonal relationship that is mutually satisfying and adaptive.	Provide consistent feedback about adaptive and maladaptive social behavior. Encourage patient to describe successful and unsuccessful relationship experiences orally or in a written journal. Assist patient in initiating or resuming a relationship with one other person. Review aspects of this relationship with patient. Reinforce patient's adaptive social responses. Evaluate with patient alternatives to maladaptive social responses.	Describing and evaluating one's behavior require taking responsibility for the behavior and its consequences. Patients need to go beyond understanding or insight to engaging in actual behavioral change. Nurse must help patient evaluate whether responses are adaptive or maladaptive. Alternatives can then be identified to further the patient's goal achievement.

Continued

/*Nursing Treatment Plan Summary*

Maladaptive Social Responses—cont'd

Short-Term Goals	Interventions	Rationale
Nursing Diagnosis: High risk for self-mutilation		
Expected Outcome: Patient will select constructive rather than self-destructive ways of coping with interpersonal anxiety.		
Patient will not engage in self-mutilation	Develop a contract with patient to notify staff when anxiety is increasing. Provide close one-on-one observation of patient when necessary to maintain safety. Remove all potentially dangerous objects from patient and environment. Provide prescribed medications.	When patient is not able to cope with anxiety, protecting patient's safety is nurse's highest priority. A contract helps patient assume responsibility and explore healthier coping responses.
Patient will describe self-mutilating episodes.	Assist patient in reviewing these events. Identify cues and triggers that precede self-mutilating behavior. Help patient explore feelings related to these episodes.	Self-mutilation is often a way of relieving extreme anxiety. Structured interpersonal support can help patient review these events.

/*Nursing Treatment Plan Summary*

Maladaptive Social Responses—cont'd

Short-Term Goals	Interventions	Rationale
Patient will describe alternatives to self-mutilating behaviors.	Suggest alternative behaviors, such as seeking interpersonal support or engaging in an adaptive anxiety-reducing activity.	Nurse can help patient review the full range of adaptive responses. Supportive but critical evaluation is necessary for behavioral change.
Patient will implement one new adaptive response when experiencing high interpersonal anxiety.	Assist patient in selecting new adaptive responses. Reinforce patient's adaptive behavior. Identify positive consequences of the adaptive responses. Discuss ways these may be generalized to other situations.	Nurse should take an active role in setting limits, examining patient behaviors, and reinforcing adaptive actions. These new learned responses can also be reviewed for their applicability to other life events.

EVALUATION

1. Has the patient become less impulsive, manipulative, or narcissistic?
2. Does the patient express satisfaction with the quality of interpersonal relationships?
3. Can the patient participate in close interpersonal relationships?
4. Does the patient verbalize recognition of positive behavioral change?

 Your Internet Connection

> **BPD Central Borderline Personality Disorder**
> www.bpdcentral.com
>
> **Mental Help NET—Personality Disorders**
> http://mentalhelp.net/poc/center_index.php?id=8
>
> **Personality Disorders Foundation**
> http://pdf.uchc.edu

■ COGNITIVE RESPONSES

Maladaptive cognitive responses include inability to make decisions, impaired memory and judgment, disorientation, misperceptions, decreased attention span, and difficulties with logical reasoning. They may occur episodically or be present continuously. Depending on the stressor, the condition may be reversible or characterized by progressive deterioration in functioning.

ASSESSMENT

Behaviors

The specific cognitive disorders to be considered include delirium and dementia. Table 17-1 describes the characteristics of delirium and dementia. Depression in elderly people is often misdiagnosed as dementia and is included in Table 17-1 for purposes of comparison.

Predisposing Factors

Cognitive responses are generally the result of a biological disruption in the functioning of the central nervous system (CNS). Factors that predispose the individual to developing cognitive disorders include the following:

1. Interference with the supply of oxygen, glucose, and other essential basic nutrients to the brain
   - Arteriosclerotic vascular changes

Table 17-1	Comparison of Delirium, Depression, and Dementia		
	DELIRIUM	**DEPRESSION**	**DEMENTIA**
Onset	Rapid (hours to days)	Rapid (weeks to months)	Gradual (years)
Course	Wide fluctuations; may continue for weeks if cause not found	May be self-limited or may become chronic without treatment	Chronic; slow but continuous decline
Level of consciousness	Fluctuates from hyperalert to difficult to arouse	Normal	Normal
Orientation	Patient is disoriented, confused	Patient may seem disoriented	Patient is disoriented, confused
Affect	Fluctuating	Sad, depressed, worried, guilty	Labile; apathy in later stages
Attention	Always impaired	Difficulty concentrating; patient may check and recheck all actions	May be intact; patient may focus on one thing for long periods
Sleep	Always disturbed	Disturbed; excess sleeping or insomnia, especially early morning waking	Usually normal
Behavior	Patient is agitated, restless	Patient may be fatigued, apathetic; may occasionally be agitated	Patient may be agitated or apathetic; may wander

From Holt J: *Am J Nurs* 93(8):32, 1993.

	DELIRIUM	DEPRESSION	DEMENTIA
Speech	Sparse or rapid; patient may be incoherent	Flat, sparse, may have outbursts; understandable	Sparse or rapid; repetitive; patient may be incoherent
Memory	Impaired, especially for recent events	Varies day to day; slow recall; often short-term deficit	Impaired, especially for recent events
Cognition	Disordered reasoning	May seem impaired	Disordered reasoning and calculation
Thought content	Incoherent, confused; delusions; stereotyped	Negative; hypochondriac, thoughts of death; paranoid	Disorganized, rich content, delusional, paranoid
Perception	Misinterpretations, illusions, hallucinations	Distorted; patient may have auditory hallucinations; negative interpretation of people and events	No change
Judgment	Poor	Poor	Poor; socially inappropriate behavior
Insight	May be present in lucid moments	May be impaired	Absent
Performance on mental status exams	Poor but variable; improves during lucid moments and with recovery	Memory impaired; calculation, drawing, following directions usually not impaired; frequent "I don't know" answers	Consistently poor; progressively worsens; patient attempts to answer all questions

- Transient ischemic attacks
- Cerebral hemorrhage
- Multiple small brain infarcts
2. Degeneration associated with aging
3. Collection of toxic substances in brain tissue
4. Alzheimer's disease
5. Human immunodeficiency virus (HIV)
6. Chronic liver disease
7. Chronic renal disease
8. Vitamin deficiencies (particularly thiamine)
9. Malnutrition
10. Genetic abnormalities

Major psychiatric disorders, such as schizophrenia, bipolar disorder, anxiety disorders, and depression, may also influence cognitive functioning.

Precipitating Stressors

Any major assault on the brain is likely to result in a disruption in cognitive functioning. Categories of stressors include the following:

1. Hypoxias
2. Metabolic disorders, including hypothyroidism, hyperthyroidism, hypoglycemia, hypopituitarism, and adrenal disease
3. Toxicity and infection
4. Adverse response to medication
5. Structural changes in the brain, such as tumors or traumas
6. Sensory underload or overload

Coping Mechanisms

The way an individual copes emotionally with maladaptive cognitive responses is greatly influenced by past life experience. A person who has developed many coping mechanisms that have been effective in the past is better able to handle the onset of a cognitive problem than a person who already has coping problems. Usual coping mechanisms may be exaggerated as the person tries to adapt to loss of cognitive ability.

Because the basic behavioral disruption in delirium is altered awareness, which reflects a severe biological disturbance in the brain, psychological coping mechanisms are not generally used. For this reason the nurse must protect the patient from harm and substitute for the person's own coping mechanisms by constantly reorienting the patient and reinforcing reality.

Behaviors that may represent attempts by the person with dementia to cope with loss of cognitive ability may include suspiciousness, hostility, joking, depression, seductiveness, and withdrawal. Ego defense mechanisms that may be observed in patients with cognitive impairment include the following:

- Regression
- Denial
- Compensation

NURSING DIAGNOSIS

Most disorders that result in some degree of cognitive impairment are physiological in origin. Therefore the nurse must consider the patient's physical needs and the psychosocial behavioral problems. A thorough nursing diagnosis reflects all these influences on the patient's behavior. If the patient's cognitive disability interferes with participation in the treatment planning process, it may be necessary to involve a significant other in the formation of the nursing diagnosis.

The box on page 310 presents the primary and related nursing diagnoses for maladaptive cognitive responses. A complete nursing assessment would include all of the patient's nursing care needs, and many additional nursing diagnoses would be identified.

NANDA NURSING DIAGNOSES

Related to Maladaptive Cognitive Responses

Anxiety
Caregiver role strain
Communication, Impaired verbal
Confusion, Acute or chronic*
Health maintenance, Ineffective
Home maintenance, Impaired
Injury, Risk for
Noncompliance
Role performance, Ineffective
Self-care deficit (specify: bathing/hygiene, dressing/grooming, feeding, toileting)
Sensory perception, Disturbed (specify: visual, auditory, kinesthetic, gustatory, tactile, olfactory)
Sleep pattern, Disturbed
Social interaction, Impaired
Thought processes, Disturbed*
Trauma, Risk for

From North American Nursing Diagnosis Association: NANDA nursing diagnoses: definitions and classification 2005-2006, *Philadelphia, 2005, The Association.*
*Primary nursing diagnosis for maladaptive cognitive responses.

Related Medical Diagnoses

The box on pages 311-313 describes mental disorders that result in maladaptive cognitive responses.

OUTCOME IDENTIFICATION

The expected outcome for a patient with maladaptive cognitive responses is as follows:

The patient will achieve optimal cognitive functioning.

DSM-IV-TR MEDICAL DIAGNOSES

Related to Cognitive Responses

DSM-IV-TR Diagnosis	*Essential Features*
Delirium (general criteria) (to be applied to all other categories of delirium)	Disturbed consciousness accompanied by a cognitive change that cannot be accounted for by a dementia. Impaired ability to focus, sustain, or shift attention. Cognitive changes, including impaired recent memory, disorientation to time or place, language disturbance, or perceptual disturbance. Develops over a short time; tends to fluctuate during the course of the day.
Delirium caused by a general medical condition	Evidence that the cognitive disturbance is the direct result of a general medical condition.
Substance-induced delirium	Evidence of substance intoxication or withdrawal, medication side effects, or toxin exposure judged to be related to the delirium.
Delirium with multiple etiologies	Evidence of multiple causes for the delirium.
Dementia (general criteria to be applied to all other categories of dementia)	Development of multiple cognitive deficits, including memory impairment and at least one of the following: aphasia, apraxia, agnosia, or disturbed executive functioning (ability to think abstractly and plan, initiate, sequence, monitor, and stop complex behavior). Must cause severe impairment in social or occupational functioning.

Modified from American Psychiatric Association: Diagnostic and statistical manual of mental disorders, *ed 4, text revision (DSM-IV-TR), Washington, DC, 2000, The Association.*   *Continued*

DSM-IV-TR MEDICAL DIAGNOSES

Related to Cognitive Responses—cont'd

DSM-IV-TR Diagnosis	*Essential Features*
Dementia of the Alzheimer's type	Gradual onset with continuing cognitive decline. All other causes of dementia must be ruled out.
Vascular dementia	Focal neurological signs and symptoms or laboratory evidence of cerebrovascular disease that are judged to be related to the dementia.
Dementia caused by other general medical conditions	Evidence that the general medical condition (e.g., HIV, traumatic brain injury, Parkinson's disease, Huntington's disease, Pick's disease, Creutzfeldt-Jakob disease, normal-pressure hydrocephalus, hypothyroidism, brain tumor, vitamin B_{12} deficiency) is etiologically related to the dementia.
Substance-induced persisting dementia	Deficits do not occur exclusively during a delirium and persist beyond the usual duration of substance intoxication or withdrawal. Evidence that the deficits are related to persisting effects of substance use (e.g., drug of abuse, medication).
Dementia caused by multiple etiologies	Evidence that the dementia has more than one etiology.
Amnestic disorder (general criteria)	Development of memory disorder evidenced by impaired ability to learn new information or to recall previously learned information. Disturbance causes significant impairment in social or occupational functioning and represents a significant decline from a previous level of functioning. Does not occur exclusively during the course of delirium or dementia.

DSM-IV-TR MEDICAL DIAGNOSES	
Related to Cognitive Responses—cont'd	
DSM-IV-TR Diagnosis	*Essential Features*
Amnestic disorder caused by a general medical condition	Evidence that the disturbance is directly related to a general medical condition (including physical trauma).
Substance-induced persisting amnestic disorder	Evidence that the memory disturbance is etiologically related to the persisting effects of substance use (e.g., drug abuse, medication).

PLANNING

A **Family Education Plan for helping the family of a patient with maladaptive cognitive response** is presented on pages 314-315.

IMPLEMENTATION

Intervening in Delirium

Nursing interventions for the patient with delirium include the following:

1. **Meeting physiological needs**
   - Maintain nutrition and fluid/electrolyte balance.
   - Use nursing measures such as back rub, warm milk, and soothing conversation to promote sleep. Sedatives may be contraindicated until the cause of the delirium has been found.
2. **Intervening in perceptual disturbances** (e.g., hallucinations)
   - Keep light on in room to minimize shadows.
   - Ensure safety by placing the patient in a room with security screens and removing excess furniture.

FAMILY EDUCATION PLAN

HELPING A FAMILY MEMBER WITH MALADAPTIVE COGNITIVE RESPONSES

Content	Instructional Activities	Evaluation
Explain possible causes of maladaptive cognitive responses.	Describe predisposing factors and precipitating stressors that may lead to impaired cognition; provide printed reference materials.	Family identifies possible causes of patient's disorders.
Define and describe orientation to time, place, and person.	Define three spheres of orientation; role-play interpersonal responses to disorientation.	Family identifies disorientation and provides reorientation.
Describe relationship of cognitive functioning level to ability to communicate.	Describe impact of maladaptive cognitive responses on communication; demonstrate effective communication techniques; videotape and discuss return demonstration.	Family adjusts communication approaches to patient's ability to interact.
Describe effect of maladaptive cognitive responses on self-care behaviors.	Describe usual progression of gain or loss of self-care ability related to nature of disorder; encourage learner to assist in providing care to patient; provide written instructional materials.	Family assists with activities of daily living as required by patient's level of biopsychosocial functioning.

FAMILY EDUCATION PLAN

HELPING A FAMILY MEMBER WITH MALADAPTIVE COGNITIVE RESPONSES—CONT'D

Content	Instructional Activities	Evaluation
Refer to community resources.	Provide a list of community resources; arrange to meet with staff members of selected community programs; visit meetings of selected programs.	Family describes various programs that provide services relevant to patient's and family's needs and will contact appropriate programs when needed.

 NURSE **ALERT**

Restraining a delirious patient to maintain an intravenous line may increase agitation. Use restraint only when absolutely necessary, and never leave a restrained delirious patient alone.

- Provide one-to-one nursing care if needed to maintain orientation.
- Reorient frequently to time, place, and person.

3. **Communication**
   - Give clear messages.
   - Avoid giving choices.
   - Use simple, direct statements.

4. **Patient education**
   - Provide information regarding cause of delirium.
   - Teach the patient and family about prescribed treatment.
   - Inform about prevention of future episodes.
   - Refer to community health nursing agency if further education or nursing intervention is required.

Intervening in Dementia

Nursing interventions for the patient with dementia include the following:

1. **Orientation**
   - Mark room clearly with the patient's name.
   - Encourage the patient to keep personal possessions in room.
   - Use a night light.
   - Provide clocks and calendars.
   - Provide newspapers and discuss them with the patient.
   - Orient verbally at frequent intervals.
2. **Communication**
   - Introduce yourself.
   - Show unconditional positive regard for the patient.
   - Use clear, concise verbal communication.
   - Modulate voice.
   - Avoid pronouns.
   - Use yes/no questions.
   - Request one thing at a time.
   - Ensure that verbal agrees with nonverbal communication.
   - Learn about the patient's past life.
   - Provide a sense of sheltered freedom.
3. **Reinforcing coping mechanisms**
4. **Decreasing wandering.** Map the patient's behavior to identify conditions under which the behavior occurs, and intervene preventively.

5. **Decreasing agitation**
   - Explain expectations clearly.
   - Offer choices if the patient can handle them.
   - Provide a schedule of activities.
   - Avoid power struggles. If the patient refuses a request, leave and return in a few minutes.
   - Involve the patient in care whenever possible.
6. **Treating pharmacologically.** Donepezil (Aricept), galantamine (Reminyl), and rivastigmine (Exelon) delay progression of Alzheimer's disease. Tacrine (Cognex), a fourth agent, is used only occasionally because of liver toxicity problems. Olanzapine (Zyprexa) can control the agitation associated with dementia and Alzheimer's disease.
7. **Involving family members**
8. **Using community resources**

Nursing interventions with patients who have maladaptive cognitive responses are provided in the **Nursing Treatment Plan Summary** below and on pages 318-320.

/*Nursing Treatment Plan Summary*

Maladaptive Cognitive Responses

Nursing Diagnosis: Altered thought processes

Expected Outcome: Patient will achieve optimal cognitive functioning.

Short-Term Goals	Interventions	Rationale
Patient will meet basic biological needs.	Maintain adequate nutrition; monitor fluid intake and output; monitor vital signs.	Basic biological integrity is necessary for survival.

Continued

/*Nursing Treatment Plan Summary*

Maladaptive Cognitive Responses—cont'd

Short-Term Goals	Interventions	Rationale
Patient will be safe from injury.	Provide opportunities for rest and stimulation. Assist with ambulation if necessary. Assist with hygiene activities as needed. Assess sensory and perceptual functioning. Provide access to eyeglasses, hearing aids, canes, walkers, etc., if needed. Observe and correct safety hazards (e.g., obstacles, slippery floors, open flames, inadequate lighting). Supervise medications if necessary. Protect from injury during periods of agitation with one-to-one nursing care; use restraints only if absolutely necessary.	Interventions related to survival are given high priority for nursing intervention. Maladaptive cognitive responses usually involve sensory and perceptual disorders that can endanger patient's safety.

/*Nursing Treatment Plan Summary*

Maladaptive Cognitive Responses—cont'd

Short-Term Goals	Interventions	Rationale
Patient will experience an optimal level of self-esteem.	Provide reality orientation. Establish a trusting relationship. Encourage independence. Identify interests and skills; provide opportunities to use them. Give honest praise for accomplishments. Use therapeutic communication techniques to help patient communicate thoughts and feelings.	Cognitive impairment is a threat to self-esteem; a positive nurse-patient relationship can assist patient to express fears and feel secure in the environment; recognition of accomplishments also raises self-esteem.

Continued

Nursing Treatment Plan Summary

Maladaptive Cognitive Responses—cont'd		
Short-Term Goals	**Interventions**	**Rationale**
Patient will maintain positive interpersonal relationships.	Initiate contact with significant others. Encourage patient to interact with others; involve in group activities. Teach family and patient about nature of the problem and recommended health care plan. Allow significant others to assist in patient care. Meet with significant others regularly and provide them with an opportunity to talk. Involve patient and family in discharge planning.	Caring relationships with others promote a positive self-concept; communication by significant others can often be understood more easily than that of strangers; family and friends can provide help in knowing patient's habits and preferences; involvement of significant others in caregiving often helps them cope with the stress of patient's health problem.

EVALUATION

1. Was the assessment complete enough to correctly identify the problem?
2. Were the goals individualized for this patient?
3. Was enough time allowed for goal achievement?
4. Did the nurse have the skills needed to carry out the identified interventions?
5. Did environmental factors affect goal achievement?
6. Did additional stressors affect the patient's ability to cope?
7. Was the goal achievable for this patient?
8. What alternative approaches could be tried?

 Your Internet Connection

Alzheimer's Association
www.alz.org

Alzheimer's Disease Education and Referral Center
www.alzheimers.org

Alzheimer's Research Forum
www.alzforum.org/home.asp

Alzwell Caregiver Support
www.alzwell.com

Dementia Research Centre
www.dementia.ion.ucl.ac.uk

Family Caregiver Alliance
www.caregiver.org

CHEMICALLY MEDIATED RESPONSES AND SUBSTANCE-RELATED DISORDERS

■ CHEMICALLY MEDIATED RESPONSES

Although there is a continuum from occasional drug or alcohol use to frequent use to abuse and dependence, not everyone who uses substances becomes an abuser, and every abuser does not become dependent.

- **Substance abuse** refers to continued use even after problems occur.
- **Substance dependence** indicates a severe condition, usually considered a disease.
- **Addiction** generally refers to the psychosocial behaviors related to substance dependence. The terms *addiction* and *dependence* are often used interchangeably.
- **Dual diagnosis** refers to the coexistence of substance abuse and psychiatric disorders within the same person.
- **Withdrawal symptoms** result from a biological need for the drug.
- **Tolerance** means that it takes increasing amounts of the substance to produce the expected effect. Withdrawal symptoms and tolerance are signs of *physical* dependence.

Abused substances include alcohol, opiates, prescription medications, psychotomimetics, cocaine, marijuana, and inhalants. A serious and growing problem in substance abuse is the rapidly increasing use of more than one substance simultaneously or sequentially.

ASSESSMENT

Behaviors

Behaviors that indicate the presence of a substance abuse problem can be assessed by using a screening tool:

- Box 18-1 presents the Brief Drug Abuse Screening Tool (B-DAST)

BOX **18-1**

Brief Drug Abuse Screening Test (B-DAST)

Instructions: The following questions concern information about your involvement in and abuse of drugs. Drug abuse refers to (1) the use of prescribed or over-the-counter drugs in excess of the directions and (2) any nonmedical use of drugs. Carefully read each statement and decide whether your answer is yes or no. Then circle the appropriate response.

Yes   No   1. Have you used drugs other than those required for medical reasons?

Yes   No   2. Have you abused prescription drugs?

Yes   No   3. Do you abuse more than one drug at a time?

Yes   No   4. Can you get through the week without using drugs (other than those required for medical reasons)?*

Yes   No   5. Are you always able to stop using drugs when you want to?*

Yes   No   6. Have you had blackouts or flashbacks as a result of drug use?

Yes   No   7. Do you ever feel bad about your drug abuse?

From Skinner HA: Addict Behav 7(4):363, 1982.
*Items 4 and 5 are scored in the "no" or false direction.

Continued

BOX **18-1**

Brief Drug Abuse Screening Test (B-DAST)— cont'd

Yes No   8. Does your spouse (or parents) ever complain about your involvement with drugs?

Yes No   9. Has drug abuse ever created problems between you and your spouse?

Yes No   10. Have you ever lost friends because of your use of drugs?

Yes No   11. Have you ever neglected your family or missed work because of your use of drugs?

Yes No   12. Have you ever been in trouble at work because of drug abuse?

Yes No   13. Have you ever lost a job because of drug abuse?

Yes No   14. Have you gotten into fights when under the influence of drugs?

Yes No   15. Have you engaged in illegal activities in order to obtain drugs?

Yes No   16. Have you ever been arrested for possession of illegal drugs?

Yes No   17. Have you ever experienced withdrawal symptoms as a result of heavy drug intake?

Yes No   18. Have you had medical problems as a result of your drug use (e.g., memory loss, hepatitis, convulsions, bleeding)?

Yes No   19. Have you ever gone to anyone for help for a drug problem?

Yes No   20. Have you ever been involved in a treatment program specifically related to drug use?

BOX **18-2**

The CAGE Questionnaire

- Have you ever felt you ought to **C**ut down on your drinking?
- Have people **A**nnoyed you by criticizing your drinking?
- Have you ever felt bad or **G**uilty about your drinking?
- Have you ever had a drink first thing in the morning to steady your nerves or get rid of a hangover (**E**ye opener)?

Scoring: 1 "yes" answer calls for further inquiry.

From Ewing JA: Detecting alcoholism: the CAGE Questionnaire, JAMA 252:1905, 1984.

- Box 18-2 presents the CAGE screening tool for alcoholism.

Individuals who abuse substances face significant risks because of their lifestyle. Accidents and violence occur frequently. Self-neglect contributes to physical, mental, and dental disease. Intravenous drug users and their partners are at high risk for infections with blood-borne pathogens, including HIV and hepatitis B virus (HBV).

Those who are *dually diagnosed* have both a substance use and a psychiatric disorder. Their substance use (1) may be causing the psychopathology; (2) may be secondary to the psychopathology as they self-medicate with substances to treat the symptoms of their mental disorder, use substances to enhance symptoms, or use substances to counter the side effects of medications they are taking for their psychiatric disorder; or (3) may be coincidental and not related to the mental disorder.

Table 18-1 summarizes the behaviors associated with substance abuse including signs and symptoms of use, dependence, overdose, and withdrawal.

Table 18-1 Characteristics of Substances of Abuse

SUBSTANCE/COMMON STREET NAMES	ROUTE/PHYSICAL DEPENDENCE/ PSYCHOLOGICAL DEPENDENCE	SIGNS AND SYMPTOMS	SPECIAL CONSIDERATIONS/ CONSEQUENCE OF USE
Depressants			
Alcohol Booze, brew, juice, spirits	Ingestion Yes/yes	*Use* Depression of major brain functions such as mood, cognition, attention, concentration, insight, judgment, memory, affect, emotional rapport in interpersonal relationships; extent of depression is dose dependent and ranges from lethargy through anesthesia and death; psychomotor impairment, increased reaction time, interruption of hand-eye coordination, motor ataxia; nystagmus, decreased rapid eye movement sleep leading to more dreams and sometimes nightmares.	Chronic alcohol use leads to serious disruptions in most organ systems: malnutrition and dehydration; vitamin deficiency leading to Wernicke's encephalopathy and alcoholic amnestic syndrome; impaired liver function, including hepatitis and cirrhosis; esophagitis, gastritis, pancreatitis; osteoporosis; anemia; peripheral neuropathy; impaired pulmonary function; cardiomyopathy; myopathy; disrupted immune system; brain damage.
Barbiturates Barbs, beans, black beauties, blue angels, candy, downers, goof balls, G.B., nebbies, reds, sleepers, yellow jackets, yellows	Ingestion, injection Yes/yes		
Benzodiazepines Downers	Ingestion, injection Yes/yes		

SUBSTANCE/COMMON STREET NAMES	ROUTE/PHYSICAL DEPENDENCE/ PSYCHOLOGICAL DEPENDENCE	SIGNS AND SYMPTOMS	SPECIAL CONSIDERATIONS/ CONSEQUENCE OF USE
Depressants—cont'd		*Overdose* Unconsciousness, coma, respiratory depression, death. *Withdrawal* General depressant withdrawal syndrome; tremors, agitation, anxiety, diaphoresis, increased pulse and blood pressure, sleep disturbances, hallucinosis, seizures, delusions, delirium tremens. *High-dose sedative-hypnotic withdrawal:* short-acting sedative hypnotics (including alcohol) symptoms begin several hours to 1 day after the last dose and peak after 24-36 hours.	High susceptibility to other dependencies. Dependence on barbiturates and benzodiazepines may develop insidiously; users may underreport actual amount taken because of guilt about multiple prescriptions and abuse.

Continued

Table 18-1	Characteristics of Substances of Abuse—cont'd		
SUBSTANCE/COMMON STREET NAMES	**ROUTE/PHYSICAL DEPENDENCE/ PSYCHOLOGICAL DEPENDENCE**	**SIGNS AND SYMPTOMS**	**SPECIAL CONSIDERATIONS/ CONSEQUENCE OF USE**
Depressants—cont'd		Long-acting sedative hypnotics: symptoms peak after 5-8 days. *Low-dose sedative-hypnotic withdrawal:* usually transient "symptom rebound" effects (anxiety, insomnia) for 1-2 weeks. May have more severe symptoms: perceptual hyperacusis, psychosis, cerebellar dysfunction, seizures *Postacute (protracted) withdrawal:* irritability, anxiety, insomnia, mood instability may occur for months.	

Substance/Common Street Names	Route/Physical Dependence/ Psychological Dependence	Signs and Symptoms	Special Considerations/ Consequence of Use
Stimulants			
Amphetamines A, AMT, bam, bennies, crystal, diet pills, dolls, eye openers, lid poppers, pep pills, purple hearts, speed, uppers, wake-ups	Ingestion, injection Yes/yes	*Use* Sudden rush of euphoria, abrupt awakening, increased energy, talkativeness, elation; agitation, hyperactivity, irritability, grandiosity, pressured speech; diaphoresis, anorexia, weight loss, insomnia, increased temperature/blood	Certain amphetamines prescribed for attention deficit hyperactivity disorder in children because of a paradoxical depressant action; may be used alternately with depressants. Cocaine use may lead to multiple physical problems:
Cocaine Bernice, bernies, big C, blow, C, charlie, coke, dust, girl, heaven, jay, lady, nose candy, nose powder, snow, sugar, white lady; crack = conan, freebase, rock,	Inhalation, smoking, injection, topical Yes/yes	pressure/pulse, tachycardia, ectopic heart beats, chest pain, urinary retention, constipation, dry mouth. *High-dose:* slurred, rapid, incoherent speech; stereotypical movements, ataxic gait, teeth grinding, illogical thought processes, headache, nausea, vomiting.	destruction of the nasal septum related to snorting; coronary artery vasoconstriction; seizures; cerebrovascular accidents; transient ischemic episodes; sudden death related to respiratory arrest and myocardial infarction.

Continued

Table 18-1	Characteristics of Substances of Abuse—cont'd		
SUBSTANCE/COMMON STREET NAMES	ROUTE/PHYSICAL DEPENDENCE/ PSYCHOLOGICAL DEPENDENCE	SIGNS AND SYMPTOMS	SPECIAL CONSIDERATIONS/ CONSEQUENCE OF USE
Stimulants—cont'd			
toke, white cloud, white tornado		*Toxic psychosis:* paranoid delusions in clear sensorium; auditory, visual, or tactile hallucinations; extremely labile mood, unprovoked violence. **Overdose** Seizures, cardiac arrhythmias, coronary artery spasms, myocardial infarction, marked increase in blood pressure and temperature; can lead to cardiovascular shock and death.	Intravenous use of stimulants may lead to the serious physical consequences described under Opiates.

Substance/Common Street Names	Route/Physical Dependence/ Psychological Dependence	Signs and Symptoms	Special Considerations/ Consequence of Use
Stimulants—cont'd		*Withdrawal* *Acute withdrawal (after periods of frequent high-dose use):* intense and unpleasant feelings of depression and fatigue, and sometimes suicidal ideation. Otherwise: milder symptoms of depression, anxiety, anhedonia, sleep disturbance, increased appetite, and psychomotor retardation; decrease steadily over several weeks. Sometimes user stops stimulants purposely to decrease tolerance, decreasing amount needed to "get high."	

Continued

Table 18-1	Characteristics of Substances of Abuse—cont'd		
SUBSTANCE/COMMON STREET NAMES	ROUTE/PHYSICAL DEPENDENCE/ PSYCHOLOGICAL DEPENDENCE	SIGNS AND SYMPTOMS	SPECIAL CONSIDERATIONS/ CONSEQUENCE OF USE
Opiates			
Heroin H, horse, harry, boy, scag, shit, smack, stuff, white junk, white stuff	Injection, ingestion, inhalation Yes/yes	*Use* Euphoria, relaxation, relief from pain, nodding out (apathy, detachment from reality, impaired judgment, drowsiness), constricted pupils, nausea, constipation, slurred speech, respiratory depression.	Intravenous use leads to high risk for infection with blood-borne pathogens, such as HIV or hepatitis B; other infections (e.g., skin abscesses, phlebitis, cellulitis, and septic emboli causing pneumonia, pulmonary abscess, or subacute bacterial endocarditis) may occur as a result of lack of asepsis or contaminated substances.
Morphine	Injection Yes/yes	*Overdose* Unconsciousness, coma, respiratory depression, circulatory depression, respiratory arrest, cardiac arrest, death. Anoxia can lead to brain abscess.	
Meperidine	Ingestion, injection Yes/yes		
Codeine	Ingestion, injection Yes/yes		

SUBSTANCE/COMMON STREET NAMES	ROUTE/PHYSICAL DEPENDENCE/ PSYCHOLOGICAL DEPENDENCE	SIGNS AND SYMPTOMS	SPECIAL CONSIDERATIONS/ CONSEQUENCE OF USE
Opiates—cont'd			
Opium	Smoking, ingestion Yes/yes	*Withdrawal* *Initially*: drug craving, lacrimation, rhinorrhea, yawning, diaphoresis.	
Methadone	Ingestion Yes/yes	*In 12-72 hours*: sleep disturbances, mydriasis, anorexia, piloerection, irritability, tremor, weakness, nausea, vomiting, diarrhea, chills, fever, muscle spasms (especially in legs), flushing, spontaneous ejaculation, abdominal pain, hypertension, increased rate and depth of respirations.	

Continued

Table 18-1	Characteristics of Substances of Abuse—cont'd		
SUBSTANCE/COMMON STREET NAMES	ROUTE/PHYSICAL DEPENDENCE/ PSYCHOLOGICAL DEPENDENCE	SIGNS AND SYMPTOMS	SPECIAL CONSIDERATIONS/ CONSEQUENCE OF USE
Opiates—cont'd		*Protracted withdrawal:* hypersensitivity to sensory stimuli, paresthesias, perceptual distortions, muscle pains, twitching tremors, headache, sleep disturbances, tension, irritability, lack of energy, impaired concentration, derealization, depersonalization. May last for several months.	Chronic use leads to lack of concern about physical well-being, resulting in malnutrition and dehydration; criminal behavior may occur to acquire money for drugs.

Substance/Common Street Names	Route/Physical Dependence/Psychological Dependence	Signs and Symptoms	Special Considerations/Consequence of Use
Marijuana			
Acapulco gold, aunt mary, broccoli, dope, grass, grunt, hay, hemp, herb, J, joint, joy stick, killer weed, maryjane, pot, ragweed, reefer, smoke, weed	Smoking ingestion No/yes	**Use** Altered state of awareness, relaxation, mild euphoria, reduced inhibition, red eyes, dry mouth, increased appetite, increased pulse, decreased reflexes; panic reaction. **Overdose** Toxic psychosis. **Withdrawal** No acute symptoms, but irritability and difficulty sleeping may last for 1-2 days.	Pulmonary problems; interference with reproductive hormones; may cause fetal abnormalities.

Continued

Table 18-1	Characteristics of Substances of Abuse—cont'd		
SUBSTANCE/COMMON STREET NAMES	ROUTE/PHYSICAL DEPENDENCE/ PSYCHOLOGICAL DEPENDENCE	SIGNS AND SYMPTOMS	SPECIAL CONSIDERATIONS/ CONSEQUENCE OF USE
Hallucinogens			
Acid, LSD, DMT, mescaline, MDMA (Ecstacy) big D, blotter, blue heaven, cap, D, deeda, flash, L, mellow yellows, microdots, paper acid, sugar, ticket, yello	Ingestion, smoking No/no	*Use* Distorted perceptions and hallucinations in presence of a clear sensorium; distortions of time and space, illusions, depersonalization, mystical experiences, heightened sense of awareness; extreme mood lability; tremor, dizziness, piloerection, paresthesias, synesthesia, nausea and vomiting; increased temperature, pulse, blood pressure, and salivation; panic reaction, "bad trip."	Flashbacks may last for several months; permanent psychosis may occur.

SUBSTANCE/COMMON STREET NAMES	ROUTE/PHYSICAL DEPENDENCE/ PSYCHOLOGICAL DEPENDENCE	SIGNS AND SYMPTOMS	SPECIAL CONSIDERATIONS/ CONSEQUENCE OF USE
Hallucinogens—cont'd			
		Overdose Rare with LSD; convulsions, hyperthermia, death. *Withdrawal* None.	
Phencyclidine (PCP) Angel dust, DOA, dust, elephant, hog, peace pill, supergrass, tic tac	Smoking, ingestion No/no	*Use* Intensely psychotic experience characterized by bizarre perceptions, confusion, disorientation, euphoria, hallucinations, paranoia, grandiosity, agitation; anesthesia; apparent enhancement of strength and	If flashbacks occur, they are mild and usually not disturbing.

Continued

Table 18-1	Characteristics of Substances of Abuse—cont'd	
SUBSTANCE/COMMON STREET NAMES	ROUTE/PHYSICAL DEPENDENCE/ PSYCHOLOGICAL DEPENDENCE	SIGNS AND SYMPTOMS	SPECIAL CONSIDERATIONS/ CONSEQUENCE OF USE
Phencyclidine (PCP)–cont'd		endurance, rage reactions; may be agitated and hyperactive with tendency toward violence or catatonic and withdrawn, or vacillate between the two conditions; red, dry skin; dilated pupils, nystagmus, ataxia, hypertension, rigidity, seizures. **Overdose** Seizures, coma, death. **Withdrawal** None.	

Substance/Common Street Names	Route/Physical Dependence/Psychological Dependence	Signs and Symptoms	Special Considerations/Consequence of Use
Inhalants			
Gasoline, glue, aerosol sprays, paint thinner, rush, bolt, huffing, bagging, sniffing	Inhalation Yes/Yes	*Use* *Psychological:* belligerence, assaultive behavior, apathy, impaired judgment. *Physical:* dizziness, nystagmus, incoordination, slurred speech, unsteady gait, depressed reflexes, tremor, blurred vision, euphoria, anorexia. *Overdose* Lethargy, stupor/coma, respiratory arrest, cardiac arrhythmia.	Death from inhalants can occur in different ways: Sudden death is caused by cardiac arrhythmia—sometimes this happens the first time the person uses inhalants. Suicide may be a result of impaired judgment. Injury under the influence of inhalants may be caused by a feeling of invulnerability.

Continued

Table 18-1	Characteristics of Substances of Abuse—cont'd		
SUBSTANCE/COMMON STREET NAMES	ROUTE/PHYSICAL DEPENDENCE/ PSYCHOLOGICAL DEPENDENCE	SIGNS AND SYMPTOMS	SPECIAL CONSIDERATIONS/ CONSEQUENCE OF USE
Inhalants--cont'd			
		Withdrawal Symptoms similar to alcohol withdrawal.	Burns and frostbite can also be caused by these chemicals. Permanent cognitive impairment may require an individual to reside in structured setting.
Nicotine			
Cigarettes, cigars, bidis, kreteks, pipe tobacco, snuff, chewing tobacco	Smoking, chewing, buccal Yes/yes	*Use* Feelings of pleasure, increased alertness, enhanced mental performance; increased heart rate and blood pressure; restricts blood flow to heart muscle.	Smoking by pregnant women contributes to low birth weight, increased incidence of stillborn and premature babies.

SUBSTANCE/COMMON STREET NAMES	ROUTE/PHYSICAL DEPENDENCE/ PSYCHOLOGICAL DEPENDENCE	SIGNS AND SYMPTOMS	SPECIAL CONSIDERATIONS/ CONSEQUENCE OF USE
Nicotine—cont'd		*Overdose* N/A *Withdrawal* Anger, anxiety, depressed mood, difficulty concentrating, subsiding within 3-4 weeks; increased appetite and craving for nicotine may persist for months.	

Predisposing Factors

1. **Biological factors**
   - Familial tendency, especially for alcohol abuse
   - Altered alcohol metabolism resulting in an uncomfortable physiological response
   - Variants of the DRD2 gene, which appears to be associated with the transmission of alcoholism
2. **Psychological factors**
   - Anxious or depressive personality types
   - Low self-esteem often related to childhood abuse
   - Overlearned, maladaptive habit
   - Pleasure seeking and pain avoidance
   - Family traits, including lack of stability, lack of positive role models, lack of trust, inability to treat children as individuals, and parental addiction
3. **Sociocultural factors**
   - Availability and social acceptability of drug use
   - Societal ambivalence about or use or abuse of various substances, such as tobacco, alcohol, and marijuana
   - Cultural attitudes, values, norms, and sanctions
   - Nationality, ethnicity, and religion
   - Poverty with associated family instability and limited opportunities

Precipitating Stressors

Withdrawal. Table 18-1 presents general behaviors related to withdrawal from substances.

Coping Mechanisms

Substance abuse represents an unsuccessful attempt to cope. Healthier defense mechanisms and other adaptive behaviors are either inadequate or have not been developed. Ego defense mechanisms typically used by substance abusers include the following:
   - Denial of the problem
   - Rationalization

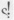 NURSE **ALERT**

A serious and potentially life-threatening alcohol withdrawal disorder is *alcohol withdrawal delirium,* formerly known as *delirium tremens* (DTs). It usually occurs on the second or third day after the last drink has been taken and ends 48 to 72 hours after onset. Behaviors include the following:

- Tremor
- Anxiety
- Paranoid delusions
- Visual hallucinations
- Disorientation
- Elevated temperature
- Tachycardia
- Tachypnea
- Hyperpnea
- Vomiting
- Diarrhea
- Diaphoresis

 NURSE **ALERT**

Another serious behavioral manifestation that may result from alcohol withdrawal is *grand mal convulsions*. These do not usually recur once alcohol withdrawal is completed.

A person can predict the severity and duration of withdrawal symptoms by using the following three rules of thumb:

1. The longer the time between last use and appearance of withdrawal symptoms, and the longer these symptoms last, the less intense they will be.
2. The longer the half-life of the drug, the longer withdrawal symptoms will last.
3. The longer the half-life of the drug, the less intense the withdrawal symptoms will be.

♩ NURSE **ALERT**

Substance use during *pregnancy* can result in the development of fetal alcohol syndrome or the birth of an addicted infant. Women should remain drug and alcohol free during pregnancy.

- Projection of responsibility for the behavior
- Minimization of the amount of alcohol or drug used

NURSING DIAGNOSIS

Individuals who have substance abuse problems also tend to develop multiple physical problems, particularly if the substance abuse problem is severe. The complete plan of nursing care would include diagnosis of all the patient's nursing care needs. The box on page 345 presents the primary and related NANDA nursing diagnoses for maladaptive chemically mediated responses.

Related Medical Diagnoses

Medical diagnoses related to maladaptive chemically mediated responses are based on the specific substance involved. The box on page 346 describes these diagnoses.

OUTCOME IDENTIFICATION

The expected outcome for a patient with substance-related withdrawal follows:

The patient will overcome addiction safely and with a minimum of discomfort.

NANDA NURSING DIAGNOSES

Related to Maladaptive Chemically Mediated Responses

Anxiety
Communication, Impaired verbal
Confusion, Acute*
Coping, Ineffective*
Family processes, Dysfunctional: alcoholism*
Hopelessness
Injury, Risk for
Noncompliance
Nutrition, Imbalanced
Parenting, Impaired
Powerlessness
Self-care deficit
Self-esteem, Chronic or Situational low
Sensory perception, Disturbed*
Sexual dysfunction
Sleep pattern, Disturbed
Spiritual distress
Spiritual distress, Risk for
Therapeutic regimen management, Ineffective: individuals or families
Thought processes, Disturbed
Violence, Risk for

From North American Nursing Diagnosis Association: NANDA nursing diagnoses: definitions and classification 2005-2006, *Philadelphia, 2005, The Association.*
Primary nursing diagnosis for chemically mediated responses.

The expected outcome for a patient with substance-related dependence follows:

The patient will abstain from using all mood-altering chemicals.

PLANNING

A **Patient Education Plan for preventing substance abuse** is presented on page 347.

DSM-IV-TR MEDICAL DIAGNOSES

Related to Maladaptive Chemically Mediated Responses

DSM-IV-TR Diagnosis	*Essential Features**
Substance dependence	Maladaptive pattern of substance use, characterized by any three of the following within 12 months: tolerance; withdrawal; using more of the substance or using for longer than planned; persistent desire but unsuccessful efforts to cut down or control use; much time spent in efforts to obtain, use, or recover from use; interference with social, occupational, or recreational activities; continued use despite knowledge of use-related recurrent physical or psychological problems.
Substance abuse	Maladaptive pattern of substance use, characterized by one or more of the following within 12 months: recurrent use resulting in failure to meet role obligations, recurrent use in physically hazardous situations, recurrent use-related legal problems, continued use despite persistent or recurrent use-related social or interpersonal problems. Has never met the criteria for dependence for the class of substance.

Modified from American Psychiatric Association: Diagnostic and statistical manual of mental disorders, ed 4, text revision (DSM-IV-TR), Washington, DC, 2000, The Association.
*A single set of essential features has been developed for substance dependence and for substance abuse. The essential features of intoxication and withdrawal vary according to the substance and are listed in Table 18-1.

PATIENT EDUCATION PLAN

PREVENTING SUBSTANCE ABUSE

Content	Instructional Activities	Evaluation
Elicit perceptions of substance use.	Lead group discussion about chemical use and experience with it. Correct misperceptions.	Patient describes accurate information about substance use.
Demonstrate negative effects of substance abuse.	Show films of physical and psychological effects of substance abuse. Provide written materials.	Patient identifies and describes physical and psychological effects of substance abuse.
Provide interaction with peer who has abused chemicals.	Initiate small group discussion with peer group member who has abused substances and quit because of negative experiences.	Patient compares and contrasts advantages and disadvantages of using mind-altering substances.
Obtain agreement to abstain from use of mind-altering substances.	Discuss future plans for refusing abused chemicals if offered.	Patient verbally agrees to abstain from using mind-altering substances.

 IMPLEMENTATION

 NURSE **ALERT**

Withdrawal from dependence on alcohol or drugs may result in life-threatening physical symptoms. The nurse should be familiar with the withdrawal symptoms presented in Table 18-1 and provide appropriate supportive interventions. Any unexpected behaviors or unanticipated worsening of the patient's condition should be reported to the physician promptly.

Biological Interventions

Intervening in Withdrawal

- Substances with potentially *life-threatening* courses of withdrawal include alcohol, barbiturates, and benzodiazepines.
- Withdrawal from opiates and stimulants can be extremely uncomfortable but is generally not dangerous, although a patient may become suicidal during the acute phase of cocaine withdrawal.
- Withdrawal from the general depressants, opiates, and stimulants is treated by gradual tapering of a drug in the same classification and treatment with symptom-specific medication.
- No identified acute withdrawal pattern is associated with marijuana, hallucinogens, or PCP.

Intervening in Toxic Psychosis. Acute toxic psychosis may result from ingestion of hallucinogens or PCP. Hallucinogen users need interpersonal intervention with constant reassurance. PCP users respond poorly to interpersonal stimulation and need to be kept in a quiet, protected environment. These patients may be terrified by the disturbances in perception that result from use of these drugs. They may act impulsively out of fear and harm themselves. Adequate staff should be available to manage this impulse behavior.

♩ NURSE **ALERT**

Unanticipated serious physiological distress in a patient who is a known or suspected substance abuser may be a sign of overdose. The nurse should be familiar with the behaviors associated with overdose of frequently abused substances. If overdose is suspected, the physician should be notified immediately.

Intervening to Maintain Abstinence. Maintaining abstinence from abused substances is one of the most difficult issues in working with patients who have substance-related disorders. In treatment for addictions, mild levels of anxiety and depression can generate motivation for change. Therefore these symptoms should not be treated with medication unless they significantly interfere with the patient's functioning and participation in the treatment plan.

A number of pharmacological therapies can help patients decrease cravings and maintain abstinence:

1. Disulfiram (Antabuse)
2. Naltrexone (Trexan)
3. Nalmefene
4. Opiate agonists, including methadone and LAAM
5. Calcium acetyl homotaurinate (acamprosate)

⚕ NURSE **ALERT**

Disulfiram (Antabuse) sensitizes alcoholic patients to alcohol. Ingestion of alcohol while taking disulfiram can lead to serious physical symptoms, possibly resulting in death. Symptoms include severe headache, nausea and vomiting, flushing, hypotension, tachycardia, dyspnea, diaphoresis, chest pain, palpitations, dizziness, and confusion. It can also lead to respiratory and cardiac collapse, unconsciousness, convulsions, and death.

The patient must be educated about the potential consequences of drinking while taking this drug. Patient education should also include the provision of a written list of alcohol-containing preparations to be avoided, including cough medicines, rubbing compounds, vinegars, aftershave lotions, and some mouthwashes. Drinking must be avoided for 14 days after disulfiram has been taken.

NURSE **ALERT**

Naltrexone (Trexan) is the first drug approved by the FDA for the treatment of alcohol dependence in more than 40 years. It blocks the euphoric effects of alcohol in the brain and promises new hope for substance abusers.

 NURSE **ALERT**

Nalmefene is a newer opioid antagonist that is structurally similar to naltrexone but with a number of pharmacological advances for the treatment of alcohol dependence. These include no dose-dependent association with toxic effects to the liver, greater oral bioavailability, longer duration of antagonist action, and more complete binding with opioid receptor subtypes that are thought to reinforce drinking. It is effective in preventing relapse to heavy drinking and has few side effects.

 NURSE **ALERT**

Acamprosate is a new drug to help prevent relapse in alcoholism. It has no sedative, antianxiety, muscle relaxant, or antidepressant properties and produces no withdrawal symptoms. Acamprosate appears to work by lowering the activity of receptors for the excitatory neurotransmitter glutamate.

Psychological and Social Interventions

Motivational counseling is one of the newer approaches to treatment. Five basic principles are used with this approach:

- *Express empathy through reflective listening.* This communicates respect for and acceptance of patients and their feelings. It also establishes a safe and open environment that helps in examining issues and exploring personal reasons for change.

- *Develop discrepancy between patients' goals or values and their current behavior.* Focus the patient's attention on how current behavior differs from behavior described as ideal or desired.
- *Avoid argument and direct confrontation.* Trying to convince a patient that a problem exists or that change is needed could precipitate even more resistance. Arguments can rapidly degenerate into a power struggle and do not enhance motivation for beneficial change.
- *Roll with resistance.* Resistance is a signal that the patient views the situation differently. There are four types of resistance: arguing, interrupting, denying, or ignoring. The clinician's job is to ask questions in a way that helps the patient to understand and work through resistance.
- *Support self-efficacy.* This requires the clinician to recognize the patient's strengths and bring these to the forefront whenever possible. It involves supporting hope, optimism, and the feasibility of accomplishing change.

Cognitive-behavioral approaches are aimed at improving self-control and social skills in order to reduce drinking. Self-control strategies include goal-setting, self-monitoring, functional analysis of drinking antecedents, and learning alternative coping skills.

Social skills training focuses on learning skills for forming and maintaining interpersonal relationships, assertiveness, and drink refusal.

Contingency management is another behavioral approach that has been successfully applied in many substance abuse treatment programs. In this strategy, rewards (often in the form of vouchers that can be exchanged for desired items) are given for adaptive behavior (such as compliance with treatment or negative urine tests).

Behavioral contracting also is a useful approach. It involves creating a written agreement with the patient that specifies targeted patient behavior and consequences.

Other social interventions can include efforts to assist the person to find **non-drug-using social supports** in the community. **Family counseling** and **self-help groups** such as Alcoholics Anonymous (AA) may be particularly helpful.

Nursing interventions with the substance-abusing patient are summarized in the **Nursing Treatment Plan Summary** on this page and pages 353-355.

/ *Nursing Treatment Plan Summary*

Maladaptive Chemically Mediated Responses

Nursing Diagnosis: Ineffective individual coping

Expected Outcome: Patient will abstain from using all mood-altering chemicals.

Short-Term Goals	Interventions	Rationale
Patient will substitute healthy coping responses for substance-abusing behavior.	Confront patient with substance-abusing behavior and its consequences. Assist patient to identify substance abuse problem. Involve patient in describing situations that lead to substance-abusing behavior. Consistently offer support and the expectation that patient does have the strength to overcome the problem.	Motivation for change is related to recognition of a problem that is upsetting to the individual. Identification of predisposing factors and precipitating stressors must precede planning for more adaptive behavioral responses.

/*Nursing Treatment Plan Summary*

Maladaptive Chemically Mediated Responses—cont'd

Short-Term Goals	Interventions	Rationale
Patient will assume responsibility for behavior.	Encourage patient to agree to participate in a treatment program. Develop with patient a written contract for behavioral change that is signed by patient and nurse. Assist patient to identify and adopt healthier coping responses.	Denial and rationalization are dysfunctional coping mechanisms that can interfere with recovery. Personal commitment enhances the likelihood of successful abstinence.
Patient will identify and use social support systems.	Identify and assess social support systems available to patient. Provide support to significant others. Educate patient and significant others about the substance abuse problem and available resources. Refer patient to appropriate resources and provide support until patient is involved in the program.	Substance abusers are often dependent and socially isolated people who use drugs to gain confidence in social situations. Substance-abusing behavior alienates significant others, thus increasing the person's isolation.

Continued

/*Nursing Treatment Plan Summary*

Maladaptive Chemically Mediated Responses—cont'd

Short-Term Goals	Interventions	Rationale
		It is difficult to manipulate people who have participated in the same behaviors. Social support systems must be readily available over time and acceptable to patient.

Nursing Diagnosis: Altered thought processes

Expected Outcome: Patient will overcome addiction safely and with a minimum of discomfort.

Short-Term Goals	Interventions	Rationale
Patient will withdraw from dependence on the abused substance.	Provide supportive physical care: vital signs, nutrition, hydration, seizure precautions. Administer medication according to detoxification schedule.	Detoxification of the physically dependent person can be dangerous and is always uncomfortable. Patient's physical safety must receive high priority for nursing intervention.

/Nursing Treatment Plan Summary

Maladaptive Chemically Mediated Responses— cont'd

Short-Term Goals	Interventions	Rationale
Patient will be oriented to time, place, person, and situation.	Assess orientation frequently; orient patient if needed; place a clock and calendar where patient can see them.	Cognitive function is usually affected by addiction; disorientation is frightening.
Patient will report symptoms of withdrawal.	Observe carefully for withdrawal symptoms and report suspected withdrawal immediately.	Withdrawal symptoms provide powerful motivation for continued substance abuse; judgment may be impaired by substance use.
Patient will correctly interpret environmental stimuli.	Explain all nursing interventions; assign consistent staff; keep soft light on in room; avoid loud noises; encourage trusted family and friends to stay with patient.	Sensory and perceptual alterations related to use of drugs or alcohol are frightening; consistency reduces need to interpret stimuli.
Patient will recognize and talk about hallucinations or delusions.	Observe for response to internal stimuli; encourage patient to describe hallucinations or delusions; explain relationship of these experiences to withdrawal from addictive substances.	Assisting patient to identify delusional or hallucinatory experiences and relate them to withdrawal is reassuring.

Interventions with Dually Diagnosed Patients

The dually diagnosed patient needs treatment for both disorders. The best treatment is an integrated one that combines pharmacological, psychosocial, and supportive services. Because both mental illness and substance abuse are chronic, relapsing conditions, the course of treatment can be expected to take considerable time. Table 18-2 describes stages of treatment and related goals and interventions for working with the dually diagnosed patient.

Table 18-2	Treatment Stages, Goals, and Interventions for Dually Diagnosed Patients	
TREATMENT STAGE	**SUGGESTED GOALS**	**SUGGESTED INTERVENTIONS**
Engagement	Development of working relationship between patient and nurse	Intervene in crises; assist with practical living problems; establish rapport with family members; demonstrate caring and support; listen actively.
Persuasion	Patient acceptance of having a substance abuse problem and the need for active change strategies	Help to analyze pros and cons of substance use; educate patient and family; arrange peer group discussions; expose patient to "double-trouble" self-help groups; adjust medication; persuade patient of need to comply with medication regimen.

Table 18-2	Treatment Stages, Goals, and Interventions for Dually Diagnosed Patients—cont'd	
TREATMENT STAGE	SUGGESTED GOALS	SUGGESTED INTERVENTIONS
Active treatment	Abstinence from substance use and compliance with medication regimen	Assist to change thinking patterns, friends, habits, behaviors, and living situations as necessary to support goals; teach social skills; encourage to develop positive social supports through double-trouble self-help groups; enlist family support of changes; monitor urine and breath for substances; offer disulfiram.
Relapse prevention	Absence or minimization of return to substance abuse	Reinforce abstinence, compliance, and behavioral changes; identify risk factors and help to practice preventive strategies; encourage continued involvement in double-trouble groups; continued laboratory monitoring.

₵ NURSE **ALERT**

Because most abused drugs cross the placental barrier, women should be counseled about the possible effects of substance use during pregnancy. The safest pregnancy is one in which the mother is totally drug and alcohol free, with one exception: for pregnant women addicted to heroin, methadone maintenance is safer for the fetus than acute opiate detoxification.

EVALUATION

1. Has the patient been able to progress significantly toward achieving the stated goals?
2. Can the patient usually communicate without being defensive?
3. Is the patient able to react appropriately, managing the demands of daily life without use of a drug?
4. Is the patient actively involved in a variety of activities, using external social and activity resources?
5. Does the patient use internal resources to be consistently productive at work and involved in meaningful interpersonal relationships?

Your Internet Connection

Adult Children of Alcoholics
www.recovery.org/acoa/acoa.html

Alcoholics Anonymous
www.alcoholics-anonymous.org

Children of Alcoholics Foundation
www.coaf.org

Drughelp
www.drughelp.org

International Nurses Society on Addictions
www.intnsa.org

National Clearinghouse on Alcohol and Drug Information
www.health.org

National Council on Alcoholism and Drug Dependence
www.ncadd.org

National Institute on Alcohol Abuse and Alcoholism
www.niaaa.nih.gov

National Institute on Drug Abuse
www.nida.nih.gov

Recovery Works
www.addictions.org/recoveryworks

Substance Abuse & Mental Health Services Administration
www.samhsa.gov

19 | EATING REGULATION RESPONSES AND EATING DISORDERS

■ EATING REGULATION RESPONSES

Adaptive eating responses are characterized by balanced eating patterns, appropriate caloric intake, and body weight that is appropriate for height and frame. Illnesses associated with maladaptive eating regulation responses include anorexia nervosa, bulimia nervosa, and binge eating disorder. These disorders can cause biological changes, including altered metabolic rates, profound malnutrition, and possibly death.

- **Anorexia nervosa** occurs in approximately 0.5% to 3.7% of the female population, with onset often between ages 13 and 20. An estimated 1 in 10 to 20 people with anorexia is male.
- **Bulimia nervosa** is more common than anorexia, with estimates of 1% to 4% of the female population and a prevalence of 4% to 15% of female high school and college students. The age at onset is typically between ages 15 and 18. An estimated 1 in 10 people with bulimia is male.

ASSESSMENT

Patients with maladaptive eating regulation responses must receive a comprehensive nursing assessment, including complete biological, psychological, and sociocultural evaluation. A full physical examination should be performed, with particular attention to vital signs, weight for height, skin, cardiovascular system, and evidence of laxative or diuretic abuse and vomiting. A dental examination may be indicated, and it is useful to assess growth, sexual development, and general physical development indicators. A psychiatric history, substance abuse history, and family assessment are also needed.

Behaviors

Box 19-1 lists key features of anorexia nervosa and bulimia nervosa.

Binge Eating. Binge eating is the rapid consumption of large quantities of food in a discrete period although no agreement exists on exactly how many calories constitute a binge. Emphasis on the individual's perception of loss of control and perceived excessive caloric intake is more important to the nursing assessment than the total number of calories consumed during a binge. Therefore the nurse must carefully assess exactly what each person means by a binge.

Fasting or Restricting. People with anorexia often do not consume more than 500 to 700 calories a day and may ingest as few as 200, but they consider their intake adequate for their energy needs. Some individuals with anorexia may not eat for days at a time. Despite these restrictions, many anorexic people are preoccupied or obsessed with food and may do much of the family cooking.

Purging. Individuals with eating disorders may use a variety of purging behaviors, including excessive exercise, over-the-counter and prescription diuretics, diet pills, laxatives, and steroids. Many patients engage in more than one purging behavior.

Medical and Psychiatric Complications. Almost every person with maladaptive eating regulation responses has

BOX **19-1**

Key Features of Anorexia Nervosa and Bulimia Nervosa

Anorexia Nervosa (Without Binging or Purging)	Bulimia Nervosa
Rare vomiting or diuretic/laxative abuse	Frequent vomiting or diuretic/laxative abuse
More severe weight loss	Less weight loss
Slightly younger	Slightly older
More introverted	More extroverted
Hunger denied	Hunger experienced
Eating behavior may be considered normal and source of esteem	Eating behavior considered foreign and source of distress
Sexually inactive	More sexually active
Obsessional and perfectionist features predominate	Avoidant, dependent, or borderline features and obsessional features
Death from starvation (or suicide in chronically ill patients)	Death from hypokalemia or suicide
Amenorrhea	Menses irregular or absent
More favorable prognosis	Less favorable prognosis
Fewer behavioral abnormalities (increase with severity)	Stealing, drug and alcohol abuse, self-mutilation, and other behavioral problems

some type of associated physical problem because all body systems are affected. Many patients seeking treatment for eating disorders also have evidence of other psychiatric disorders, such as depression, obsessive-compulsive disorder, substance abuse disorders, and personality disorders.

Predisposing Factors

Biological. Eating disorders appear to be familiar. First-degree female relatives of people with eating disorders are at higher risk than the general population. Concordance rates for eating disorders in monozygotic twins is 52% and in dizygotic twins 11%. A higher risk for other eating disorders and for depression also is seen in first-degree relatives of people with eating disorders, suggesting common etiological factors.

Biological models of the etiology of eating disorders focus on the appetite regulation center in the hypothalamus, which controls specific neurochemical mechanisms for feeding and satiety. Serotonin is thought to be involved in the pathophysiology of eating disorders, although these biological models are still in the developmental stage.

Environmental. A variety of environmental factors may predispose an individual to the development of an eating disorder. Early histories of patients with eating disorders are often complicated by medical and surgical illnesses, separations, family deaths, and conflicted family environments. Sexual abuse has been reported in 20% to 50% of patients with bulimia, but this rate may be similar to that found in patients with other psychiatric disorders.

Psychological. Most patients with eating disorders exhibit clusters of psychological symptoms, such as rigidity, ritualism, meticulousness, perfectionism, exactness, symmetry, greater risk avoidance and restraint, and poor impulse control. Early separation and individuation conflicts, a pervasive sense of ineffectiveness and helplessness, difficulty interpreting feelings and tolerating intense emotional states, and fear of biological or psychological maturity may predispose an individual to an eating disorder.

Sociocultural. In cultures where plumpness is either accepted or valued, eating disorders are rare. Also, the sociocultural environment for adolescents and young women in the United States places great emphasis on thinness and control over one's body as a yardstick for self-evaluation. Psychosocial predisposing factors for the development of eating disorders are summarized in Box 19-2.

BOX **19-2**

Psychosocial Predisposing Factors for the Development of Eating Disorders

Personal Factors
Weight
Puberty/maturation
Restrained eating/dieting
Body image dissatisfaction
Problems regulating affect
Depression
Perfectionism
Low self-esteem
Stress
Low resiliency/confidence
Poor coping skills
Alcohol and substance use
Sexual/physical abuse
Dating

Family Factors
Parental attitudes
Family functioning
Socioeconomic status

Peers
Attitudes about weight
Behaviors
Teasing

From Taylor C, Altman T: Psychopharm Bull *33(3):413, 1997.*

BOX **19-2**

Psychosocial Predisposing Factors for the
Development of Eating Disorders—cont'd

Culture
Media influences

Activities
Gymnastics
Professional dance
Modeling

Precipitating Stressors

Individuals with the previous predisposing factors are especially vulnerable to environmental pressures or life stressors, such as the loss of a significant other, interpersonal rejection, and failure.

Coping Mechanisms

Anorectic patients most frequently use the defense mechanism of denial in a severely maladaptive way, and they usually do not seek help on their own. The defense mechanisms used by bulimic patients include:

- Avoidance
- Denial
- Isolation of affect
- Intellectualization.

NURSING DIAGNOSIS

The box on page 366 presents the primary and related NANDA nursing diagnoses for maladaptive eating regulation

NANDA NURSING DIAGNOSES

Related to Maladaptive Eating Regulation Responses

Anxiety*
Body image, Disturbed*
Coping, Ineffective
Denial, Ineffective
Family processes, Interrupted
Fatigue
Fluid volume, Deficient
Hopelessness
Injury, Risk for
Nutrition, Imbalanced: less than body requirements or more than
body requirements*
Powerlessness*
Role performance, Ineffective
Self-esteem, Chronic or Situational low*
Self-mutilation, Risk for*
Sexual dysfunction

From North American Nursing Diagnosis Association: NANDA nursing diagnoses:
definitions and classification 2005-2006, *Philadelphia, 2005, The Association.*
*Primary nursing diagnosis for eating problems.

responses. Additional nursing problems resulting from the
eating disorder should also be identified.

Related Medical Diagnoses

The box on page 367 identifies the medical diagnoses related
to maladaptive eating regulation responses and their essential
features.

DSM-IV-TR MEDICAL DIAGNOSES

Related to Maladaptive Eating Regulation Responses

DSM-IV-TR Diagnosis	Essential Features
Anorexia nervosa	Intense fear of gaining weight, even when underweight. A disturbance in the way the body is experienced and a refusal to maintain body weight above a minimal normal weight for age and height lead to a body weight 15% below expected. In females there is also the absence of at least three consecutive menstrual cycles.
Bulimia nervosa	Recurrent episodes of binge eating with a feeling of lack of control over the eating behavior and persistent over-concern with body shape and weight. The individual also regularly engages in self-induced vomiting, use of laxatives, or rigorous dieting and fasting to counteract the effects of binge eating.
Binge eating disorder	Recurrent episodes of binging that are a cause of distress, with a feeling of lack of control over the eating behavior but without behaviors used to prevent weight gain.

Modified from American Psychiatric Association: Diagnostic and statistical manual of mental disorders, *ed 4, text revision (DSM-IV-TR), Washington, DC, 2000, The Association.*

OUTCOME IDENTIFICATION

The expected outcome for the patient with maladaptive eating regulation responses is as follows:

The patient will restore healthy eating patterns and normalize physiological parameters related to body weight and nutrition.

PLANNING

Important considerations in the planning phase of the nursing process are the choice of an inpatient, outpatient, or partial hospitalization treatment setting and the formulation of a nurse-patient contract. Box 19-3 presents clinical criteria for hospitalizing a patient with an eating disorder and is followed by a **Family Education Plan for preventing childhood eating problems** on pages 369–370.

BOX **19-3**

Clinical Criteria for Hospitalization of Patients with an Eating Disorder

Medical
Need for extensive diagnostic evaluation
Weight loss greater than 25% of body weight over 3 months
Heart rate less than 40 beats/min or greater than 110 beats/min
Temperature less than 97.0° F
Systolic blood pressure less than 70 mm Hg or marked orthostatic hypotension greater than 20 mm Hg/min standing
Serum potassium less than 2.5 mEq/L despite oral potassium replacement
Severe dehydration or vomiting blood
Concurrent somatic illnesses (such as infection)

Psychiatric
Risk of suicide or self-mutilation
Severe depression
Substance abuse
Psychosis
Family crisis
Failure to comply with treatment contract or poor motivation
Inadequate response to outpatient treatment

FAMILY EDUCATION PLAN

PREVENTING CHILDHOOD EATING PROBLEMS

Content	Instructional Activities	Evaluation
Describe self-demand feeding and its importance in healthy eating behaviors.	Explore current feeding practices of parents and understanding of healthy eating. Provide information to enhance knowledge of healthy eating behaviors.	Parents identify healthy eating behaviors and self-demand feeding and begin to explore how their relationship with food influences their children's eating.
Describe physiological and psychological signs of hunger and satiety, the meaning of both, and differences between both types.	Explore parents' own signs of hunger and satiety and also have parents describe their children's signs.	Parents keep a hunger diary to record physical and psychological signs of hunger and satiety for themselves and their children.
Describe danger of psychological hunger.	Explain the use of a hunger diary, which is a daily journal regarding signs of hunger.	Parents can distinguish between psychological and physical hunger.
Explore myths about feeding, e.g., "cleaning the plate" and "eating because other children are starving."	Describe the importance of allowing children to determine their feeding needs and the relationship of healthy eating to children's ability to differentiate between physical and psychological signs of hunger and satiety.	Parents complete homework assignment, discuss interview experiences, and describe how perpetuating myths about feeding can harm their children.

Continued

FAMILY EDUCATION PLAN

PREVENTING CHILDHOOD EATING PROBLEMS— CONT'D

Content	Instructional Activities	Evaluation
	Give homework assignment for each parent to interview three other adults about their current eating practices and memories of eating.	
Implement self-demand feeding at particular developmental stages of children.	Review the stages that children experience with eating and the potential problems they may have at each stage.	Parents discuss the developmental stages of their children and plan for implementing self-demand feeding.
Discuss parental experiences related to implementing self-demand feeding.	Review parents' expectations and experiences with implementing self-demand feeding.	Parents relate any problem with self-demand feeding. Nurse evaluates family for further education and plans for follow-up if necessary.

 IMPLEMENTATION

Empirically validated treatments for bulimia nervosa are summarized in Table 19-1.

Table 19-1	Summarizing the Evidence on Eating Disorders
DISORDER	**TREATMENT**
Bulimia nervosa (BN)	Several different classes of antidepressant drugs produced significant, short-term reductions in binge eating and purging. Manual-based cognitive-behavioral therapy (CBT) was most effective in eliminating the core features of BN; roughly half the patients receiving CBT reduced binge eating and purging; long-term maintenance of improvement was good.

From Nathan P, Gorman J: *A guide to treatments that work*, ed 2, New York, 2002, Oxford University Press.

Nursing care for a patient with an eating disorder includes the following areas of intervention:

1. Nutritional stabilization
2. Exercise monitoring
3. Cognitive behavioral interventions
4. Body image interventions
5. Family involvement
6. Group therapies
7. Medication

A **Nursing Treatment Plan Summary for patients with maladaptive eating regulation responses** is presented on page 372-375.

EVALUATION

1. Have normal eating patterns been restored?
2. Have the biological and psychological sequelae of malnutrition been corrected?

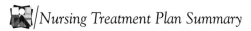/*Nursing Treatment Plan Summary*

Maladaptive Eating Regulation Responses

Nursing Diagnosis: Altered nutrition

Expected Outcome: Patient will restore healthy eating patterns and normalize physiological parameters related to body weight and nutrition.

Short-Term Goals	Interventions	Rationale
Patient will engage in treatment and acknowledge having an eating disorder.	Help patient identify maladaptive eating responses. Discuss positive and negative consequences of maladaptive eating responses. Contract with patient to engage in treatment.	First step of treatment is for patient to acknowledge the illness and see the need for help.
Patient will be able to describe a balanced diet based on the five food groups.	Complete a nutritional assessment, including eating-related behaviors and preferences. Teach, clarify, and reinforce knowledge of proper nutrition.	Knowledge of healthy nutrition is essential to establishing and maintaining adaptive eating responses.

/Nursing Treatment Plan Summary

Maladaptive Eating Regulation Responses—cont'd

Short-Term Goals	Interventions	Rationale
Patient's nutritional status will be stabilized by a specified target date.	Monitor physiological status for signs of compromised nutrition. Administer medications and somatic treatments for management of symptoms. Monitor and evaluate patient's response to somatic treatments. Implement nursing activities as specified in the program contract and protocol.	Weight stabilization must be a central and early goal for the nutritionally compromised patient. Medications may assist the appetite regulation center and neurochemical responses to feeding and satiety.
Patient will participate daily in a balanced exercise program.	Review established exercise routines. Modify exercise patterns, focusing on physical fitness rather than weight reduction. Reinforce new exercise and fitness behaviors.	Focus of a balanced exercise program should be on physical fitness rather than calorie reduction to lose weight.

Continued

Nursing Treatment Plan Summary

Maladaptive Eating Regulation Responses—cont'd

Short-Term Goals	Interventions	Rationale
Nursing Diagnosis: Body image disturbance		
Expected Outcome: Patient will express clear and accurate descriptions of body size, body boundaries, and ideal weight.		
Patient will correct body image distortions.	Modify body image misperceptions through cognitive and behavioral strategies. Use dance and movement therapies to enhance the integration of mind and body. Employ imagery and relaxation interventions to decrease anxiety related to body perceptions.	Body image distortions involve perceptions, attitudes, and behaviors that place so much emphasis on appearance that they define self-worth.
Patient will modify cognitive distortions about body weight, shape, and eating responses.	Assist patient in identifying: 1. Cues that trigger problematic eating responses and body image concerns 2. Thoughts, feelings, and assumptions associated with the specific cues	Cognitive distortions result in lowered self-esteem. Behavioral change occurs as a result of increased awareness of feelings and

/*Nursing Treatment Plan Summary*

Maladaptive Eating Regulation Responses—cont'd

Short-Term Goals	Interventions	Rationale
	3. Connections between these thoughts, feelings, and assumptions and eating regulation responses	faulty cognitions.
	4. Consequences resulting from the eating responses	
Patient will identify social support systems that reinforce accurate body perceptions and adaptive eating responses.	Include family evaluation and treatment planning process. Assess family as a system and impact of the eating disorder on family functioning. Initiate group therapy to mobilize social support and reinforce adaptive responses.	Patients with eating disorders benefit from involvement of family members and supportive group work.

3. Have the associated sociocultural and behavioral problems been resolved so that relapse does not occur?

Your Internet Connection

Academy for Eating Disorders
www.aedweb.org

American Anorexia Bulimia Association
www.aabainc.org

Eating Disorder Referral and Information Center
www.edreferral.com

National Eating Disorders Association
www.nationaleatingdisorders.org

National Eating Disorders Organization
www.kidsource.com/nedo

SEXUAL RESPONSES AND SEXUAL DISORDERS

■ SEXUAL RESPONSES

Sexuality is broadly defined as a desire for contact, warmth, tenderness, or love. It includes looking and talking; hand-holding, kissing, or self-pleasuring; and the production of mutual orgasm. Sexuality is a part of a person's total sense of self. Four aspects of sexuality are:

1. **Genetic identity**, which is a person's chromosomal gender
2. **Gender identity**, which is a person's perception of his or her own maleness or femaleness
3. **Gender role**, which is made up of the cultural role attributes of one's gender, such as expectations regarding behavior, cognitions, occupations, values, and emotional responses
4. **Sexual orientation**, which is the gender to which one is romantically attracted

The most adaptive sexual responses are seen as behaviors that meet the following criteria:

1. Between two consenting adults
2. Mutually satisfying to the individuals involved
3. Not psychologically or physically harmful to either party
4. Lacking in force or coercion
5. Conducted in private

Maladaptive sexual responses include behaviors that do not meet one or more of these criteria.

Caution must be used when attempting to label sexual behaviors as adaptive or maladaptive. For instance, sexual behavior can meet the criteria but still be unsatisfactory for an individual if altered by the impact of what society dictates as acceptable and unacceptable behavior.

ASSESSMENT

Self-Awareness of the Nurse

The most critical element in being able to counsel patients competently about sexuality is nurses' awareness of their own feelings and values. Nurses' level of self-awareness has a direct impact on their ability to intervene effectively with patients.

Behaviors

Modes of sexual expression vary greatly. Many individuals are not exclusively heterosexual or homosexual. The following are definitions of common terms:

1. **Heterosexual**—a person who is sexually attracted to members of the opposite sex
2. **Homosexual**—a person who is sexually attracted to members of the same sex
3. **Bisexual**—a person who is sexually attracted to people of both sexes
4. **Transvestite**—a person who dresses in the clothes of the opposite sex
5. **Transsexual**—a person who is genetically an anatomical male or female but who expresses, with strong conviction, that he or she has the mind of the opposite sex and seeks to change his or her sex legally and through hormonal and surgical sex reassignment

Predisposing Factors

At present, no one theory can adequately explain the process of sexual development or the factors predisposing a person to maladaptive sexual responses. Several theories have been proposed including:

1. *Biological factors*. These are initially responsible for the development of gender, that is, whether a person is genetically male or female. The person's somatotype includes chromosomes, hormones, internal and external genitalia, and gonads.

2. *Psychoanalytical view*. Freud viewed sexuality as one of the key forces of human life. He was the first theorist to believe that sexuality was developed before the onset of puberty and that a person's choice of sexual expression depended on an interplay of heredity, biology, and social factors.

3. *Behavioral view*. This perspective views sexual behavior as a measurable response, with both physiological and psychological components, to a learned stimulus or reinforcement event. The treatment of sexual problems involves processes to change behavior through direct intervention without the need to identify underlying causes or psychodynamics.

Precipitating Stressors

Sexual identity cannot be separated from a person's self-concept or body image. Therefore, when changes occur in the person's body or emotions, sexual responses change as well. Specific threats include the following:

1. Physical illness and injury
2. Psychiatric illness
3. Medications
4. HIV, acquired immunodeficiency syndrome (AIDS)
5. The aging process

Coping Mechanisms

Numerous coping mechanisms may be used in the expression of a person's sexual response, including the following:

- *Fantasy* may be used to enhance sexual experiences.
- *Denial* may be used to refuse to recognize sexual conflicts or dissatisfactions.
- *Rationalization* may be used to justify or make acceptable otherwise unacceptable sexual impulses, feelings, behaviors, or motives.
- *Withdrawal* may be used to cope with unresolved feelings about becoming vulnerable and with the resulting ambivalent feelings about intimacy.

NURSING DIAGNOSIS

The primary NANDA nursing diagnoses are altered sexuality patterns, which include lack of sexual satisfaction and con-

NANDA NURSING DIAGNOSES

Related to Variations in Sexual Response

Anxiety
Body image, Disturbed
Fear
Grieving, Dysfunctional
Grieving, Risk for dysfunctional
Health maintenance, Ineffective
Pain, Acute or Chronic
Personality identity, Disturbed
Powerlessness
Role performance, Ineffective
Self esteem, Chronic or Situational low
Sexual dysfunction*
Sexuality patterns, Ineffective*
Social interaction, Impaired
Spiritual distress
Spiritual distress, Risk for

From North American Nursing Diagnosis Association: NANDA nursing diagnoses: definitions and classification 2005-2006, Philadelphia, 2005, The Association.
***Primary nursing diagnosis for variations in sexual response.**

which includes actual physical limitations. The box on page 380 presents the primary and related NANDA diagnoses for variations in sexual response.

Related Medical Diagnoses

Many people who experience transient variations in sexual response have no medically diagnosed health problem. Patients with more severe or persistent problems are classified in one of three basic categories of DSM-IV-TR: gender identity disorders, paraphilias, and sexual dysfunctions. The box below and on pages 382-383 describes the specific medical diagnoses in each of these diagnostic classes.

DSM-IV-TR MEDICAL DIAGNOSES

Related to Variations in Sexual Response

DSM-IV-TR Diagnosis	Essential Features
Hypoactive sexual disorder	Persistent or recurrent deficit or absence of sexual fantasies and desire for sexual activity.
Sexual aversion disorder	Persistent or recurrent extreme aversion to and avoidance of all or almost all genital sexual contact with a sexual partner.
Sexual arousal disorder	Persistent or recurrent partial or complete failure to attain or maintain the physiological response of sexual activity, or persistent or recurrent lack of a subjective sense of sexual excitement and pleasure during sexual activity.
Orgasmic disorder	Persistent or recurrent delay in or absence of orgasm after a normal sexual excitement phase during sexual activity that the clinician judges to be adequate in focus, intensity, and duration, taking into account the individual's age.

Modified from American Psychiatric Association: Diagnostic and statistical manual of mental disorders, *ed 4, text revision (DSM-IV-TR), Washington, DC, 2000, The Association.* *Continued*

DSM-IV-TR MEDICAL DIAGNOSES

Related to Variations in Sexual Response—cont'd

DSM-IV-TR Diagnosis	*Essential Features*
Premature ejaculation	Persistent or recurrent ejaculation with minimal sexual stimulation, before, during, or shortly after penetration, before the individual desires it.
Dyspareunia	Recurrent or persistent genital pain before, during, or after sexual intercourse.
Vaginismus	Recurrent or persistent involuntary spasm of the musculature of the outer third of the vagina that interferes with coitus.
Sexual dysfunction caused by a general medical condition	Clinically significant sexual dysfunction etiologically related to a general medical condition.
Substance-induced sexual dysfunction	Clinically significant sexual dysfunction that developed during significant substance intoxication or withdrawal.
Exhibitionism	Persistent association, lasting at least 6 months, between intense sexual arousal, desire, acts, or fantasies and exposing one's genitals to an unsuspecting stranger.
Fetishism	Persistent association, lasting at least 6 months, between intense sexual arousal, desire, acts, or fantasies and nonliving objects (e.g., female undergarments).
Frotteurism	Persistent association, lasting at least 6 months, between intense sexual arousal, desire, acts, or fantasies and rubbing against a nonconsenting person.
Pedophilia	Persistent association, lasting at least 6 months, between intense sexual arousal, desire, acts, or fantasies and one or more children age 13 years or younger.

DSM-IV-TR MEDICAL DIAGNOSES

Related to Variations in Sexual Response—cont'd

DSM-IV-TR Diagnosis	Essential Features
Sexual masochism	Persistent association, lasting at least 6 months, between intense sexual arousal, desire, acts, or fantasies and being humiliated, beaten, bound, or otherwise being made to suffer (real or imagined).
Sexual sadism	Persistent association, lasting at least 6 months, between intense sexual arousal, desire, acts, or fantasies and the affliction of real or simulated psychological or physical suffering (including humiliation).
Voyeurism	Persistent association, lasting at least 6 months, between intense sexual arousal, desire, acts, or fantasies and observing unsuspecting people who are naked, in the act of disrobing, or engaging in sexual activity.
Transvestic fetishism	Persistent association, lasting at least 6 months, between intense sexual arousal, desire, acts, or fantasies and cross-dressing.
Gender identity disorder of childhood, adolescence, or adulthood	Persistent and intense distress about being a male or a female, with an intense desire to be the opposite sex, a preoccupation of adulthood with the activities of the opposite sex, and a repudiation of one's own anatomical structures.

OUTCOME IDENTIFICATION

The expected outcome for patients with maladaptive sexual responses is as follows:

The patient will obtain the maximal level of adaptive sexual responses to enhance or maintain health.

PLANNING

Education is the usual method of primary prevention for sexual problems and issues. A **Patient Education Plan for teaching about sexual response after an organic illness** is presented below.

PATIENT EDUCATION PLAN

SEXUAL RESPONSE AFTER AN ORGANIC ILLNESS

Content	Instructional Activities	Evaluation
Describe the variety of human sexual response patterns.	Discuss range of sexual desires, modes of expression, and techniques.	Patient identifies preferences and typical level of sexual functioning.
Define patient's primary organic problem.	Provide accurate information on disruption caused by the organic impairment.	Patient understands nature of the organic illness.
Clarify relationship between patient's organic problem and level of sexual functioning.	Reframe distorted or confused perceptions about impact of illness on sexual functioning.	Patient accurately describes the impact of illness on sexual functioning.
Identify ways to enhance patient's sexual functioning and improve interpersonal communication.	Describe additional experiences that would enhance sexual satisfaction and the relationship between patient and partner.	Patient and partner report reduced anxiety and greater satisfaction with sexual responses.

IMPLEMENTATION

Intervening in Health Education

Before engaging in either health education or counseling, nurses must examine their own values and beliefs about patients who practice sexual behavior that may be different. This can be facilitated by exploring typical myths about human sexuality held by society as listed in Table 20-1.

Table 20-1	Ten Common Myths and Facts About Human Sexuality		
MYTH	**RESULT OF MYTH**	**FACT**	
Patients become embarrassed when nurses bring up the subject of sexuality and would prefer that nurses not ask questions about sex.	If nurses believe this, they deny patients the opportunity to ask questions and clarify concerns related to sexual issues.	Patients would prefer that nurses initiate discussions of sexuality with them.	
Excessive masturbation is harmful.	Individuals often feel guilty or ashamed about masturbating; some deny themselves this experience because of uncomfortable feelings perpetuated by society.	No evidence indicates that masturbation causes physical problems. If masturbation leads to satisfaction and pleasure, it is unlikely to be a problem.	

Continued

Table 20-1	Ten Common Myths and Facts About Human Sexuality—cont'd	
MYTH	RESULT OF MYTH	FACT
Sexual fantasies about having sex with a partner other than lover or spouse indicate relationship difficulties.	Individuals may become uncomfortable about having a fantasy with a different partner. They may experience guilt feelings and view the fantasy as a sign of infidelity.	Imagining sex with a different partner is a common sexual fantasy and does not necessarily indicate desire to act out the fantasized behavior.
Sex during menstruation is unclean and harmful.	Women often view their bodies as unclean and even unfit or inferior during menstruation. Women use menstruation as an excuse to avoid intercourse rather than simply saying no without a "good reason."	Medically, menstrual flow is not harmful or dirty. If women desire, no reason exists to abstain from intercourse during menstrual flow.
Oral and anal intercourse are perverted and dangerous.	Many individuals refrain from these behaviors or indulge in them only to feel ashamed and guilty afterward.	Oral and anal intercourse are not harmful if certain precautions are taken when performing anal intercourse, such as avoiding vaginal contamination and wearing a condom to prevent disease transmission.

Table 20-1	Ten Common Myths and Facts About Human Sexuality—cont'd	
MYTH	RESULT OF MYTH	FACT
Most homosexuals molest children.	Known homosexuals are often fired from teaching jobs, and many parents will not allow their children to spend time with any homosexual.	Research shows that the adult heterosexual male poses a much greater risk to the underage child than the adult homosexual male.
Homosexuals are sick and cannot control their sexual behavior.	Homosexuals are denied jobs and are sometimes jailed for their homosexuality. Homosexual partners may have their children taken away by courts.	Most homosexuals' social and psychological adjustment is the same as that of the heterosexual majority, and objectionable sexual advances are much more likely to be made by a heterosexual (usually male to female) than a homosexual.
Because of sex education programs, most adolescents and young adults are aware of the risks of acquiring sexually transmitted diseases (STDs) and practice safe sex.	When health educators believe that young adults have adequate knowledge about STDs, they may not take the time to assess further, add to this knowledge, and correct any misconceptions.	A study of more than 500 freshmen at a large university reported that of those who had multiple partners, fewer than 50% used condoms to lower the risk of disease.

Continued

Table 20-1	Ten Common Myths and Facts About Human Sexuality—cont'd	
MYTH	**RESULT OF MYTH**	**FACT**
Advancing age means the end of sex.	Many older adults become victims of this myth not because their bodies have lost the ability to perform, but because they believe they have lost the ability to perform.	Sexually, men and women in good health can function effectively throughout their lives.
Alcohol ingestion reduces inhibitions and therefore enhances sexual enjoyment.	Many individuals use alcohol in the hope that it will increase their sexual pleasure and performance. Alcohol ingestion can also provide an excuse for engaging in sexual behaviors, e.g., "I would never have gone to bed with him if I hadn't had all that wine."	Data do not support the belief that alcohol ingestion reduces inhibitions and enhances sexual enjoyment.

Intervening in Sexual Responses in the Nurse-Patient Relationship

Feelings of sexual attraction and sexual fantasies are part of the human experience, and the nurse should address them. Two aspects of this include a nurse's sexual attraction to a patient and the patient's sexual acting out or display of seductive behaviors toward the nurse. Table 20-2 summarizes considerations in sexual responses of patients to nurses.

Table 20-2	Nursing Interventions in Sexual Responses of Patients to Nurses	
PRINCIPLE	**RATIONALE**	**NURSING INTERVENTIONS**

Goal: Maintain a professional nurse-patient relationship that will enable nurse to provide therapeutic nursing care.

| Establish a trusting relationship. | Atmosphere of trust allows for open, honest communication between patient and nurse; when this occurs, nurse can aid patient in discovering underlying issues related to patient's sexual feelings and behavior. | Express nonsexual caring and concern for patient. Be a responsible listener, especially to feelings and needs that patient may not be able to express directly. Reinforce purpose of professional, therapeutic nurse-patient relationship. |
| Be aware of own feelings and thoughts. | When aware of his or her own feelings and thoughts, the nurse will begin to understand how they influence behavior. With increased self-awareness, nurse increases effectiveness of interactions with patients. | Recognize own feelings and thoughts. Identify any specific patient interaction or behavior that influences feelings and thoughts. Identify influence of feelings and thoughts on behavior to increase effectiveness of interventions. |

Continued

Table 20-2	Nursing Interventions in Sexual Responses of Patients to Nurses—cont'd	
PRINCIPLE	**RATIONALE**	**NURSING INTERVENTIONS**
Decrease patient's inappropriate expressions of sexual feelings and behavior.	If nurse can help patient see that the sexual interactions and behavior are being expressed to an inappropriate partner (nurse), sexual acting out will usually decrease. Nurse can help patient begin to identify reasons for behavior.	Set limits on patient's sexual behavior. Use a calm, matter-of-fact approach without implying judgment. Reaffirm nonsexual caring for patient. Explore meaning of patient's feelings and behavior.
Expand patient's insight into sexual feelings and behavior.	Once patient begins to identify reasons for sexual feelings and behaviors, patient can see that nurse is not an appropriate outlet for these feelings and behaviors. Patient then can move toward a more appropriate and therapeutic relationship with nurse.	Clarify misconceptions about any feeling patient may have about nurse as possible sexual partner. Point out futile nature of patient's romantic or sexual interest. Redirect patient's energies toward appropriate health care issues.

Patients may also experience maladaptive sexual responses resulting from physical and emotional illness, sexual preference, gender identity, or dysfunctions of the sexual response cycle. A **Nursing Treatment Plan Summary** for maladaptive sexual responses is presented below and on pages 392-393.

Nursing Treatment Plan Summary

Maladaptive Sexual Response

Nursing Diagnosis: Altered sexuality pattern

Expected Outcome: Patient will obtain the maximal level of adaptive sexual responses to enhance or maintain health.

Short-Term Goals	Interventions	Rationale
Patient will describe values, beliefs, questions, and problems regarding sexuality.	Listen to sexual concerns implied and expressed. Help patient explore sexual beliefs, values, and questions. Encourage open communication between patient and partner.	An accepting therapeutic relationship will allow patients to be free to question, grow, and seek help with sexual concerns. Communicate respect, acceptance, and openness to sexual concerns.

Continued

/*Nursing Treatment Plan Summary*

Maladaptive Sexual Response—cont'd

Short-Term Goals	Interventions	Rationale
Patient will relate accurate information about sexual concerns.	Clarify sexual misinformation. Dispel myths. Provide specific education about sexual health practices, behaviors, and problems. Give professional "permission" to continue sexual behavior that is not physically or emotionally harmful. Reinforce positive attitudes of patient.	Accurate information is helpful in changing negative thoughts and attitudes about particular aspects of sexuality. It can also prevent or limit dysfunctional behavior. Giving permission allows patient to continue the behavior and alleviate anxiety about normalcy. Patient can incorporate sexual behavior in a positive and accepting self-concept.

/*Nursing Treatment Plan Summary*

Maladaptive Sexual Response—cont'd

Short-Term Goals	Interventions	Rationale
Patient will implement one new behavior to enhance sexual response.	Set clear goals with patient. Identify specific behaviors that can be carried out, focusing on enhancing self-concept, role functioning, and sexuality. Encourage relaxation techniques, redirection of attention, positional changes, and alternative ways of sexual expression as appropriate. Become familiar with sexuality therapy resources available in the community. Refer patient to a qualified sexuality therapist as needed.	Giving patient direct behavioral suggestions can help relieve a sexual problem or difficulty and is a useful intervention when the problem is of recent onset and short duration. All nurses must screen for maladaptive sexual responses and provide basic nursing care, but should refer complex problems to qualified sexuality therapists for further treatment.

EVALUATION

1. Were the nurse's own feelings and values about sexuality explored and handled appropriately in giving patient care?
2. Was the nursing assessment of the patient's sexuality complete, accurate, and done professionally?
3. Have the patient's feelings about self improved during treatment?
4. If the patient was dysfunctional, was functional ability improved or restored?
5. Was health teaching on variations in sexual expression appropriately carried out?
6. Have the patient's interpersonal relationships improved?
7. Did the patient think that the care was helpful in meeting health care goals?
8. Is referral to another health care professional or agency indicated for the patient?

Your Internet Connection

American Association of Sex Educators, Counselors and Therapists (AASECT)
www.aasect.org

Association for Gay, Lesbian and Bisexual Issues in Counseling
www.aglbic.org

The Kinsey Institute
www.kinseyinstitute.org

Sexual Health Network
www.sexualhealth.com

Sexuality Information and Education Council of the United States
www.siecus.org

Society for the Scientific Study of Sexuality (SSSS)
www.sexscience.org

■ ROLE OF THE NURSE

The nurse should be knowledgeable about psychopharmacology, but this information must be used as one part of a holistic approach to patient care. The nurse's role includes the following:

1. *Patient assessment.* Before initiation of psychopharmacological treatment, a thorough biopsychosocial evaluation must be completed, including the following:
   - Physical examination
   - Laboratory studies
   - Mental status evaluation
   - Medical and psychiatric history
   - Medication history
   - Family history

   The Medication Assessment Tool presented in Box 21-1 can be used to take a drug history.

2. *Coordination of treatment modalities.* This integrates the varied medication and nonmedication treatments. Drug interactions are of concern for patients who are prescribed multiple medications. Table 21-1 lists some of the more common interactions of psychotropic drugs and other substances.

3. *Administration of psychopharmacological agents.* This provides a professionally designed and individualized drug administration regimen.

4. *Monitoring drug effects.* This includes both desired effects

BOX **21-1**

Medication Assessment Tool

For each of the following categories of drugs taken by the patient:
- Prescribed psychiatric medications ever taken
- Prescribed nonpsychiatric medication taken in the past 6 months or taken for major medical illnesses if more than 6 months ago
- Over-the-counter (OTC) medication taken in the past 6 months

Obtain the following information from the patient and other sources:
- Name of the drug
- Reason taken
- Dates started and stopped
- Highest daily dose
- Who prescribed it?
- Was it effective?
- Side effects or adverse reactions
- Was it taken as directed?
- If not, how was it taken?
- History of drug taken by first-degree relative
- Drugs taken prescribed by others
- Supplements, herbs, essential oils, and other complementary and alternative remedies either prescribed or OTC

For each of the following categories of drugs taken by the patient:
- Alcohol
- Tobacco
- Caffeine
- Street drugs

BOX **21-1**

Medication Assessment Tool—cont'd

Obtain the following information from the patient and other sources:
- Name of substance
- Dates and schedule of use
- Summarize effects
- Adverse reactions/withdrawal symptoms
- Attempts to stop/treatments to stop
- Impact of substance on:
  - Quality of life
  - Relationships/spouse/children
  - Occupation/education
  - Health/productivity
  - Self-image
  - Expense

---

and adverse or side effects that patients may experience.

5. *Patient education.* This enables patients to take their medicines safely and effectively.

6. *Drug maintenance program.* This is designed to support the patient in aftercare settings for extended periods.

7. *Participation in interdisciplinary clinical research drug trials.* The nurse is an essential member of the team who researches the drugs used to treat patients with psychiatric disorders.

8. *Prescriptive authority.* Some psychiatric nurses who are qualified by education and experience in accordance with their state practice act are able to prescribe pharmacological agents to treat the symptoms and improve the functional status of patients with psychiatric illness.

Table 21-1	Interactions of Psychotropic Drugs and Other Substances
PSYCHOTROPIC CATEGORY	POSSIBLE INTERACTIONS

Antianxiety Agents

Benzodiazepines with

Central nervous system (CNS) depressants (alcohol, barbiturates, antipsychotics, antihistamines, cimetidine)	Potential additive CNS effects, especially sedation and decreased daytime performance
Selective serotonin reuptake inhibitors (SSRIs), disulfiram, estrogens	Increased benzodiazepine effects
Antacids, tobacco	Decreased benzodiazepine effects

Sedative-hypnotics with

CNS depressants (alcohol, antihistamines, antidepressants, narcotics, antipsychotics)	Enhancement of sedative effects; impairment of mental and physical performance; may result in lethargy, respiratory depression, coma, death
Anticoagulants (oral)*	Decreased coumarin plasma levels and effect; monitor and adjust dose of coumarin

Antidepressants

Tricyclics (TCAs) with

Monoamine oxidase inhibitors (MAOIs)*	May cause hypertensive crisis
Alcohol and other CNS depressants	Additive CNS depression; decreased TCA effect
Antihypertensives* (guanethidine, methyldopa, clonidine)	Antagonism of antihypertensive effect
Antipsychotics and anti-parkinsonians	Increased TCA effect; confusion, delirium, ileus
Anticholinergics	Additive anticholinergic effects
Antiarrhythmics (quinidine, procainamide, propranolol)	Additive antiarrhythmic effects; myocardial depression

*Potentially clinically significant.

Table 21-1	Interactions of Psychotropic Drugs and Other Substances—cont'd
PSYCHOTROPIC CATEGORY	**POSSIBLE INTERACTIONS**

Antidepressants–cont'd

Tricyclics (TCAs) with—cont'd

SSRIs*	Increased TCA serum level/ toxicity through inhibition of cytochrome P-450 system
Anticonvulsants	Decreased TCA effect; seizures
Tobacco	Decreased TCA plasma levels

SSRIs with

Clomipramine, maprotiline, bupropion, clozapine	Increased risk of seizures
MAOIs*	Serotonin syndrome
Barbiturates, benzodiazepines, narcotics	Increased CNS depression
Carbamazepine	Neurotoxicity: nausea, vomiting, vertigo, tinnitus, ataxia, lethargy, blurred vision
Aripiprazole	Fluoxetine and paroxetine lower levels
Risperidone	Fluoxetine and paroxetine may increase risperidone to toxic levels
Selegiline*	Hypertensive crisis; increased serotonergic effects; mania
St. John's wort, naratriptan, rizatriptan, sumatriptan, zolmitriptan, tramadol*	Serotonin syndrome
Haloperidol	Decreased effect of either drug
Calcium channel blockers	Neurotoxicity; dizziness, nausea, diplopia, headache
Valproate	Decreased valproate serum concentration
Cimetidine, erythromycin, isoniazid, fluconazole	Somnolence, lethargy, dizziness, blurred vision, ataxia, nausea; increased carbamazepine levels

Continued

Table 21-1	Interactions of Psychotropic Drugs and Other Substances—cont'd
PSYCHOTROPIC CATEGORY	**POSSIBLE INTERACTIONS**

Antidepressants–cont'd

SSRIs with—cont'd

Clozapine*	Avoid due to increased risk of agranulocytosis
Aripiprazole	Increased blood levels of aripiprazole
Rifampin	Decreased carbamazepine levels

Antipsychotics With

Antacids, tea, coffee, milk, fruit juice	Decreased phenothiazine effect
CNS depressants (narcotics, antianxiety drugs, alcohol, antihistamines, barbiturates)	Additive CNS depression
Anticholinergic agents (levodopa)*	Additive atropine-like side effects and increased anti-Parkinson effects
SSRIs	Increased neuroleptic serum level and extrapyramidal side effects (EPS)

Antipsychotics

Clozapine with

Carbamazepine*	Additive bone marrow suppression
Benzodiazepines*	Circulatory collapse, respiratory arrest
SSRIs*	Increased risk of seizures

*Potentially clinically significant.

♩ NURSE **ALERT**

Concurrent use of drugs, or *polypharmacy*, can enhance a specific therapeutic action, can be necessary to treat concurrent illnesses, and can counteract unwanted effects of the first drug. Unfortunately, several problems are associated with concurrent drug use, including confusion over therapeutic efficacy and side effects and development of drug interactions.

■ ANTIANXIETY AND SEDATIVE-HYPNOTIC DRUGS

Antianxiety and sedative-hypnotic drugs are divided into two categories: the benzodiazepines and the nonbenzodiazepines, which include several classes of drugs. The benzodiazepines are the most widely prescribed drugs in the world, and in the last 20 years they have almost entirely replaced the barbiturates in the treatment of anxiety and sleep disorders. Their popularity is related to their effectiveness and wide margin of safety.

Benzodiazepines

Mechanism of Action. The benzodiazepines are thought to exert their antianxiety effects through their powerful potentiation of the inhibitory neurotransmitter γ-aminobutyric acid (GABA).

Clinical Use. The benzodiazepines are frequently the drug of choice in the management of anxiety, insomnia, and stress-related conditions (Table 21-2). Most experts believe that treatment with benzodiazepines should be brief, during periods of specific stress. With supervision, however, they are often given for extended periods.

Table 21-2   Antianxiety and Sedative-Hypnotic Drugs: Benzodiazepines

Generic Name (Trade Name)	Active Metabolites	Approximate Half-Life (hr)	Usual Adult Dosage Range (mg/day)*	Preparation
Antianxiety Drugs				
Alprazolam (Xanax)	Yes (not significant)	14	1-4	PO
Chlordiazepoxide (Librium)	Yes	20-30	10-40	PO, IM
Clonazepam (Klonopin)	No	>20	0.5-10	PO, ODT
Clorazepate (Tranxene)	Yes	60	10-40	PO, SD
Diazepam (Valium)	Yes	10-60	2-40	PO, SR, IM, IV
Halazepam (Paxipam)	Yes	60	60-160	PO
Lorazepam (Ativan)	No	14	1-6	PO, IM, IV
Oxazepam (Serax)	No	9	15-120	PO
Prazepam (Centrax)	Yes	60	10-60	PO

*Dosage ranges are approximate and should be individualized for each patient.
HS, at bedtime; IM, intramuscular; IV, intravenous; ODT, orally disintegrating tablet; PO, oral tablet or capsule; SD, single dose; SR, oral slow-release tablet.

Table 21-2	Antianxiety and Sedative-Hypnotic Drugs: Benzodiazepines—cont'd			
GENERIC NAME (TRADE NAME)	ACTIVE METABOLITES	APPROXIMATE HALF-LIFE (HR)	USUAL ADULT DOSAGE RANGE (MG/DAY)*	PREPARATION
Sedative-Hypnotic Drugs				
Estazolam (ProSom)	Yes	16	1-4	HS PO
Flurazepam (Dalmane)	Yes	100	15-30	HS PO
Temazepam (Restoril)	No	8	7.5-30	HS PO
Triazolam (Halcion)	No	3	0.125-0.5	HS PO
Quazepam (Doral)	Yes	39	7.5-15	HS PO

*Dosage ranges are approximate and should be individualized for each patient.
HS, at bedtime; IM, intramuscular; IV, intravenous; ODT, orally disintegrating tablet; PO, oral tablet or capsule; SD, single dose; SR, oral slow-release tablet.

The major indications for benzodiazepine use follow:

1. Generalized anxiety disorder
2. Anxiety associated with depression
3. Sleep disorders
4. Anxiety associated with phobic disorders
5. Posttraumatic stress disorder
6. Alcohol and drug withdrawal
7. Anxiety associated with medical disease
8. Musculoskeletal relaxation
9. Seizure disorders
10. Preoperative anxiety

Adverse Reactions and Nursing Considerations. The benzodiazepines have a very high therapeutic index; thus overdoses of these drugs alone almost never cause fatalities. Side effects are common, dose related, and almost always harmless. Table 21-3 summarizes these reactions and identifies nursing considerations.

Table 21-3	Benzodiazepine Side Effects and Nursing Considerations
SIDE EFFECTS	NURSING CONSIDERATIONS*
Common	
Drowsiness, sedation	Activity helps; use caution when using machinery.
Ataxia, dizziness	Use caution with activity; prevent falls.
Feelings of detachment	Discourage social isolation.
Increased irritability or hostility	Observe, support, be alert for disinhibition.
Anterograde amnesia	Inability to recall events that occur while on drug.

*Benzodiazepines are contraindicated in patients with a history of drug or alcohol abuse.

Table 21-3	Benzodiazepine Side Effects and Nursing Considerations—cont'd
SIDE EFFECTS	**NURSING CONSIDERATIONS***

Common—cont'd

Cognitive effects with long-term use	Interference with concentration and memory of new material.
Tolerance, dependency, rebound insomnia/ anxiety	Use for short term; discontinue, using a slow taper; contraindicated with drug or alcohol abuse.

Rare

Nausea	Dose with meals; decrease dose.
Headache	Usually responds to mild analgesic.
Confusion	Decrease dose.
Gross psychomotor impairment	Dose related; decrease dose.
Depression	Decrease dose; antidepressant treatment.
Paradoxical rage reaction	Discontinue drug.

*Benzodiazepines contraindicated in patients with a history of drug or alcohol abuse.

⚕ NURSE **ALERT**

The benzodiazepines generally are not as strongly addictive as thought if their discontinuation is accomplished by gradual tapering, if they have been used for appropriate purposes, and if their use has not been complicated by the use of other substances, such as chronic use of barbiturates or alcohol. Watch particularly for the following:

- Sedation
- Ataxia
- Irritability
- Memory problems

Nonbenzodiazepines

The nonbenzodiazepines have been largely replaced by the benzodiazepines although they are used occasionally. Table 21-4 lists the nonbenzodiazepine antianxiety and sedative-hypnotic agents.

Table 21-4	Nonbenzodiazepine Antianxiety and Sedative-Hypnotic Agents	
GENERIC NAME (TRADE NAME)	**DOSE (MG/DAY)**	**HALF-LIFE (HR)**
Antianxiety Agents		
Buspirone (BuSpar)	15-60	2-5
Propranolol (Inderal)	60-160	3
Clonidine (Catapres)	0.2-0.6	6-20
Sedative-Hypnotic Agents		
Zolpidem (Ambien)	5-10	1-2.5
Zaleplon (Sonata)	5-10	1-2.5
Antihistamines (also used for sleep)		
Diphenhydramine (Benadryl)	50	Unknown
Hydroxyzine (Atarax, Vistaril)	100-300	Unknown
Antidepressant		
Trazodone (Desyrel)	50-200	4

♩ NURSE **ALERT**

> Use of barbiturates has numerous disadvantages, as follows:
> 1. Tolerance develops to the antianxiety effects of barbiturates.
> 2. They are more addictive.
> 3. They cause serious and even lethal withdrawal reactions.
> 4. They are dangerous in overdose and cause central nervous system (CNS) depression.
> 5. They have a variety of dangerous drug interactions.

■ ANTIDEPRESSANTS

The types of antidepressant drugs are tricyclics (TCAs), monoamine oxidase inhibitors (MAOIs), selective serotonin reuptake inhibitors (SSRIs), and a group of other antidepressants not in the first three classes (Table 21-5). The primary clinical indication for the use of antidepressant drugs is major depressive illness. They are also useful in the treatment of panic disorder, other anxiety disorders, and enuresis in children. Preliminary research studies suggest they are useful for attention deficit disorders in children and for bulimia and narcolepsy.

Tricyclic Antidepressants

Mechanism of Action. The TCAs appear to regulate the brain's use of the neurotransmitters norepinephrine and serotonin.

Clinical Use. With an acceptable cardiac history and an electrocardiogram (ECG) within normal limits, particularly for people more than 40 years old, TCAs are safe and effective in the treatment of acute and long-term depressive illnesses.

Table 21-5	Antidepressant Drugs

GENERIC NAME (TRADE NAME)	USUAL ADULT DAILY DOSE (MG/DAY)*	PREPARATIONS
Selective Serotonin Reuptake Inhibitors (SSRIs)		
Citalopram (Celexa)	20-40	PO, L
Escitalopram (Lexapro)	20-40	PO
Fluoxetine (Prozac)	20-60	PO, L
Fluvoxamine (Luvox)	100-200	PO
Paroxetine (Paxil)	20-50	PO, CR
Sertraline (Zoloft)	50-200	PO, L
Other New Antidepressant Drugs		
Amoxapine (Asendin)	200-300	PO
Bupropion (Wellbutrin)	150-450[†]	PO, SR
Maprotiline (Ludiomil)	50-200[†]	PO
Mirtazapine (Remeron)	15-45	PO
Serotonin antagonist and reuptake inhibitors (SARIs)		
Nefazodone (Serzone)	300-500	PO
Trazodone (Desyrel)	150-300	PO
Serotonin-norepinephrine reuptake inhibitor (SNRI)		
Venlafaxine (Effexor)	75-375	PO, XR
Tricyclic Antidepressant Drugs (TCAs)		
Tertiary (parent)		
Amitriptyline (Elavil)	150-300	PO, IM
Clomipramine (Anafranil)	100-250	PO
Doxepin (Sinequan)	150-300	PO, L
Imipramine (Tofranil)	150-300	PO
Trimipramine (Surmontil)	150-300	PO

*Dosage ranges are approximate; initiate at lower dose for most patients.
[†]Antidepressants with a ceiling dose due to dose-related seizures.
CR, controlled release; IM, intramuscular; L, Oral liquid; PO, oral tablet/capsule; SR, sustained release; TS, transdermal system patch; XR, extended release.

Table 21-5	Antidepressant Drugs—cont'd	
Generic Name (Trade Name)	**Usual Adult Daily Dose (mg/day)**	**Preparations**
Secondary (metabolite)		
Desipramine (Norpramin)	150-300	PO, L
Nortriptyline (Pamelor)	50-150	PO, L
Protriptyline (Vivactil)	15-60	PO
Tetracyclics		
Amoxapine (Asendin)	150-400	PO
Maprotiline (Ludiomil)	150-225	PO
Monoamine Oxidase Inhibitors (MAOIs)		
Isocarboxazid (Marplan)	20-60	PO
Phenelzine (Nardil)	45-90	PO
Selegiline (Eldepryl, Emsam)	20-50	PO, TS
Tranylcypromine (Parnate)	20-60	PO

Adverse Reactions and Nursing Considerations. The nurse should know the common side effects of the antidepressants and be aware of toxic effects and their treatment. These drugs cause sedation and anticholinergic side effects, such as dry mouth, blurred vision, constipation, urinary retention, orthostatic hypotension, temporary confusion, tachycardia, and photosensitivity.

Most of these are common, short-term side effects and can be minimized with a decrease in dose. Toxic side effects include confusion, poor concentration, hallucinations, delirium, seizures, respiratory depression, tachycardia, bradycardia, and coma.

NURSE **ALERT**

1. Antidepressants have a 3- to 4-week delay before therapeutic response.
2. They have no known long-term adverse effects.
3. Tolerance to therapeutic effects does not develop.
4. Persistent side effects can often be minimized by a small decrease in dose.
5. They do not cause physical addiction or psychological dependence.
6. They do not cause euphoria; thus they have no abuse potential.
7. Many can be conveniently given once a day.

 NURSE **ALERT**

1. Tricyclic antidepressants can be lethal in overdose.
2. They also can have dangerous cardiac side effects, requiring EKGs in all children and adults with cardiac problems.

Monoamine Oxidase Inhibitors (MAOIs)

Mechanism of Action. MAOIs block monoamine oxidase in the brain and the rest of the body. By blocking MAO in the brain, less norepinephrine is metabolized, thus increasing its availability in the synapse.

Clinical Use. MAOIs are very effective antidepressant and antipanic drugs that have been underused and overly feared. Because of the potential for hypertensive crisis when tyramine-containing foods and certain medicines are taken concomitantly with these drugs, careful health teaching of a reliable patient is important. Box 21-2 outlines dietary restrictions with MAOI therapy.

BOX 21-2

Dietary Restrictions: 1 Day Before, During, and 2 to 6 Weeks After MAOI Therapy

Food and Beverages to Avoid

Cheese, especially aged or matured
Fermented or aged protein (meat or fish)
Pickled or smoked fish
Chianti and vermouth wines, tap (draft) beer
Yeast or protein extracts
Fava or broad bean pods
Liver, sausages, pepperoni, salami, canned ham
Spoiled or overripe fruit
Banana peel, sauerkraut

Food and Beverages to Be Consumed in Moderation

Chocolate
Yogurt, sour cream, cottage and cream cheese
Clear spirits and white wine
Avocado, raspberries
New Zealand spinach
Soy sauce
Aspartame, monosodium glutamate

Drugs to Avoid

Most other antidepressant drugs
Other MAOIs
Nasal and sinus decongestants
Allergy and hay fever remedies
Narcotics, especially meperidine
Asthma remedies
Local anesthetics with epinephrine
Weight-reducing pills, pep pills, stimulants
Cocaine, amphetamines
Other medications without first checking with clinician

Continued

BOX **21-2**

Dietary Restrictions: 1 Day Before, During, and 2 to 6 Weeks After MAOI Therapy—cont'd

Medications That May Need Dose Decreased
Insulin and oral hypoglycemics
Oral anticoagulants
Thiazide diuretics
Anticholinergic agents
Muscle relaxants

Adverse Reactions and Nursing Considerations. Side effects of MAOIs include lightheadedness, constipation, sexual dysfunction, muscle twitching, drowsiness, dry mouth, fluid retention, insomnia, urinary hesitancy, and weight gain. Box 21-3 lists signs and treatment of hypertensive crisis during MAOI therapy.

BOX **21-3**

Signs and Treatment of Hypertensive Crisis During MAOI Therapy

Warning Signs
Increased blood pressure, palpitations, frequent
  headaches

Symptoms of Hypertensive Crisis
Sudden elevation of blood pressure
Explosive headache, occipital that may radiate frontally
Head and face flushed and feel "full"
Palpitations, chest pain
Sweating, fever
Nausea, vomiting
Dilated pupils
Photophobia
Intracranial bleeding

BOX **21-3**

Signs and Treatment of Hypertensive Crisis During MAOI Therapy—cont'd

Treatment

Hold next MAOI dose.

Do not have patient lie down (elevates blood pressure in head).

Administer intramuscular chlorpromazine, 100 mg; repeat if necessary (mechanism of action: blocks norepinephrine).

Administer intravenous phentolamine slowly in 5-mg doses (mechanism of action: binds with norepinephrine receptor sites, blocking norepinephrine).

Manage fever with external cooling techniques.

Evaluate diet, adherence to regimen, and education.

♩ NURSE **ALERT**

1. MAOIs may be lethal in overdose.
2. Dietary restrictions must begin several days before taking the medication, be maintained while taking the medication, and be continued for 2 weeks after discontinuing therapy.
3. These drugs are nonaddicting.
4. Tolerance does not develop for therapeutic effects.
5. MAOIs decrease the body's ability to use vitamin B_6; thus supplements may be necessary.

Selective Serotonin Reuptake Inhibitors

Mechanism of Action. The SSRIs inhibit the reuptake of serotonin at the presynaptic membrane. Thus these drugs promote the neurotransmission of serotonin in the brain. One of the newer antidepressants, venlafaxine, raises the levels of serotonin and norepinephrine. Thus it has a broad spectrum of activity and is called a nonselective reuptake inhibitor.

Clinical Use. SSRIs not only represent a new approach to the treatment of depression and other disorders (e.g., panic disorder, obsessive-compulsive disorder) but also may provide a safer treatment option than other antidepressants because they are relatively safe in overdose. In addition, the SSRIs have a safer side effect profile than the TCAs and MAOIs.

Adverse Reactions and Nursing Considerations. The SSRIs have antidepressant effects comparable to the other classes of antidepressant drugs but without significant anti-cholinergic, cardiovascular, and sedative side effects. The most common side effects include nausea, diarrhea, insomnia, dry mouth, nervousness, headache, sexual dysfunction, drowsiness, dizziness, and sweating. Most of these are short-term side effects and can be minimized by supportive measures, titrating the dose, or changing the medication schedule (Table 21-6).

■ MOOD-STABILIZING DRUGS

Table 21-7 lists the major mood-stabilizing drugs.

Lithium

Mechanism of Action. Lithium is a naturally occurring salt, and the exact mechanism of action is not fully understood. Many neurotransmitter functions are altered.

Table 21-6	Antidepressant Side Effects and Nursing Considerations
SIDE EFFECT	NURSING CONSIDERATIONS

Anticholinergic Side Effects

Blurred vision	Temporary; avoid hazardous tasks.
Dry mouth	Encourage fluids, frequent rinses, sugar-free hard candy and gums; check for mouth sores.
Constipation	Increase fluids, dietary fiber and roughage, exercise; monitor bowel habits; use stool softeners and laxatives only if necessary.
Tachycardia	Temporary, usually not significant (except with coronary artery disease), but can be frightening; eliminate caffeine; β-blockers might help; supportive therapy.
Urinary retention	Encourage fluids and frequent voiding; monitor voiding patterns; bethanechol; catheterize.
Cognitive dysfunction	Temporary; avoid hazardous tasks, adjust lifestyle; offer supportive therapy.
Cytochrome P-450 inhibition*	SSRIs inhibit the liver isoenzyme cytochrome P-450, which is instrumental in the metabolism of a variety of drugs (TCAs, trazodone, barbiturates, most benzodiazepines, carbamazepine, narcotics, neuroleptics, phenytoin, valproate, verapamil). This effect can be potentially life threatening because it increases serum concentrations as well as therapeutic and toxic effects of these drugs.

NOTE: Always educate the patient and use the techniques in this table. Consider decreasing or dividing drug dose. Change drug only if necessary.

*Potentially life-threatening.

BP, Blood pressure; ECG, electrocardiogram; GI, gastrointestinal; HS, at bedtime; 5-HT, serotonin; MAOIs, monoamine oxidase inhibitors. SSRIs, selective serotonin reuptake inhibitors; TCAs, tricyclic antidepressants.   *Continued*

416

Unit Two   Clinical Care

Table 21-6	Antidepressant Side Effects and Nursing Considerations—cont'd
SIDE EFFECT	**NURSING CONSIDERATIONS**
Dizziness/ lightheadedness	Dangle feet; adequate hydration, elastic stockings; protect from falls.
ECG changes	Careful cardiac history; pretreatment ECG for patients more than age 40 and children; ST segment depression, T wave flattened or inverted, QRS prolongation; worsening of intraventricular conduction problems; do not use if there is recent myocardial infarction or bundle-branch block.
Ejaculatory dysfunction	Dose after sexual intercourse, not immediately before.
GI disturbances (nausea, diarrhea)	Take with meals or at HS; adjust diet if indicated.
Hallucinations, delusions, activation of schizophrenic or manic psychosis	Change to another antidepressant class of drug, initiate antipsychotics or mood stabilizers if appropriate.
Hypertensive crisis*	See Box 21-3.
Hypotension	Frequent BP; hydrate; elastic stockings; may need to change drug. For postural hypotension: lying and standing BP, gradual change of positions, protect from falls.
Insomnia	Dose as early in the day as possible; sleep hygiene, decrease evening activities; eliminate caffeine; relaxation techniques; sedative-hypnotic therapy.
Memory dysfunction	Temporary; encourage concentration, make lists, provide social support, adjust lifestyle.
Perspiration (excessive)	Frequent change of clothes, cotton/linen clothing, good hygiene; increase fluids.
Priapism	Change dose, change drug.

Table 21-6	Antidepressant Side Effects and Nursing Considerations—cont'd
SIDE EFFECT	**NURSING CONSIDERATIONS**
Psychomotor activation	Take drug in morning rather than at HS, adjust lifestyle.
Sedation/drowsiness	Administer drug at HS, avoid hazardous tasks.
Serotonin syndrome (SS)*	SS is a life-threatening emergency resulting from excess central nervous system 5-HT caused by combining 5-HT-enhancing drugs or administering SSRIs too close to the discontinuation of MAOIs. Symptoms are confusion, disorientation, mania, restlessness/agitation, myoclonus, hyperreflexia, diaphoresis, shivering, tremor, diarrhea, nausea, ataxia, headache. Discontinue all serotonergic drugs immediately; anticonvulsants for seizures; serotonin antagonist drugs may help; clonazepam for myoclonus, lorazepam for restlessness/agitation, other symptomatic care as indicated; do not reintroduce serotonin drugs.
Sexual dysfunction	Dose after sexual intercourse, use lubricant if vaginal dryness is present; give antidotes such as sildenafil, bupropion, or bethanechol.
Tachycardia	See anticholinergic side effects.
TCA withdrawal syndrome	Symptoms: malaise, muscle aches, chills, nausea, dizziness, coryza; when discontinuing drug, taper over several days or weeks.
Tremors	Temporary; adjust lifestyle if indicated.
Weight gain	Increase exercise; reduced calorie diet if indicated; may need to change class of drug.

Table 21-7 Mood Stabilizing Drugs

Drug Class, Generic Name (Trade Name)	Half-Life (hr)	*Usual Adult Dose (mg/day)	Preparations
Antimania			
Lithium (Eskalith, Lithobid)	18-36	600-2400	PO, CR, SR
Lithium citrate	18-36	600-2400	L/S
Anticonvulsants			
Valproic acid (Depakene); valproate (Depacon), divalproex (Depakote)	9-16	15-60 mg/kg/day	PO, L/S, ER, IM
Lamotrigine (Lamictal)	25-32	300-500	PO, Ch
Carbamazepine (Tegretol)	25-65	200-1600	PO, Ch
Gabapentin (Neurontin)	5-7	900-3600+	PO
Oxcarbazepine (Trileptal)	2-9	600-2400	PO, S
Topiramate (Topamax)	20-30	200-400	PO
Tiagabine (Gabitril)	7-9	4-32	PO
Atypical Antipsychotic			
Olanzapine (Zyprexa)	27	15-20	PO

*The dosage range is approximate and must be individualized for each patient.
Ch, Chewable tablets; CR, controlled release; ER, sustained release; IM, injection; L/S, liquid/syrup; PO, oral tablets or capsules; S, suspension; SR, slow release.

BOX **21-4**

Lithium Levels

Common Causes for Increased Lithium Levels
1. Decreased sodium intake
2. Diuretic therapy
3. Decreased renal functioning
4. Fluid and electrolyte loss: sweating, diarrhea, dehydration
5. Medical illness
6. Overdose
7. Nonsteroidal antiinflammatory drug therapy

Ways to Maintain Stable Lithium Levels
1. Stabilize dosing schedule by dividing doses or using sustained-release capsules.
2. Maintain adequate dietary sodium and fluid intake (2-3 quarts/day).
3. Replace fluid and electrolytes during exercise or gastrointestinal illness.
4. Monitor signs and symptoms of lithium side effects and toxicity.
5. If patients forget a dose, they may take it if they missed dosing time by 2 hours; if longer than 2 hours, skip that dose and take the next dose; never double-up doses.

Clinical Use. Acute episodes of mania and hypomania and recurrent bipolar illness are the most common indications for lithium treatment. Other disorders with an affective component, such as recurrent unipolar depression, schizoaffective disorder, catatonia, rage reactions, and alcoholism, are sometimes effectively treated with lithium, especially when they are periodic or cyclical.

Adverse Reactions and Nursing Considerations.
Patients can take lithium for many years. They must be
taught the common causes for an increase in lithium level
and ways to stabilize a therapeutic level (Box 21-4). Lithium
side effects include fine hand tremor, fatigue, headache,
mental dullness, lethargy, polyuria, polydipsia, gastric irrita-
tion, mild nausea, vomiting, diarrhea, acne, ECG changes,
and weight gain.

Signs of lithium toxicity are related to lithium levels and
include anorexia, nausea, vomiting, diarrhea, coarse hand
tremor, twitching, lethargy, dysarthria, ataxia, fever, irregular
vital signs, seizures, and coma.

Anticonvulsants

A number of anticonvulsant drugs have been used
successfully to treat bipolar illness (Table 21-7) including:

- Divalproex (Depakote)—well tolerated in general;
  side effects include anorexia, nausea, vomiting,
  diarrhea, tremor, sedation, ataxia, weight gain, and,
  very rarely, pancreatitis and hepatic dysfunction,
  which necessitate regular laboratory studies.
- Lamotrigine (Lamictal)—useful in delaying onset of
  mood episodes in patients receiving standard
  treatment for acute mood episodes in bipolar disorder.
- Carbamazepine (Tegretol)—has a variety of effects in
  the brain that help to stabilize mood. Side effects
  include drowsiness, dizziness, ataxia, blurred vision,
  nausea, vomiting, and skin rash. A rare but serious
  problem is agranulocytosis; thus blood levels and
  complete blood counts are monitored frequently.

Atypical Antipsychotics

The atypical antipsychotic olanzapine (Zyprexa) has FDA
approval for the treatment of acute mania. Evidence indicates that it has mild antidepressant properties as well. Data
suggest that olanzapine will prove useful in preventing sub-

sequent cycles of mania or depression as a maintenance treatment.

The atypical antipsychotic aripiprazole (Abilify) has also been approved for the treatment of bipolar disorder, and numerous reports have indicated that other atypical antipsychotic drugs are also effective in the treatment of this disorder. The prescription of these drugs, particularly in combination with other mood stabilizers, is becoming common clinical practice. However, their precise mechanism of action for this disorder is unclear.

⚕ NURSE **ALERT**

1. Lithium toxicity is a life-threatening emergency.
2. Blood levels must be monitored frequently.
3. Treatment failures may occur.
4. Lithium can also be combined with other antidepressants.
5. Patients need careful education about maintenance of lithium levels.
6. Lithium is sometimes used to augment the efficacy of other antidepressants

---

▪ ANTIPSYCHOTIC DRUGS

Mechanism of Action

Antipsychotic drugs are dopamine antagonists and block dopamine receptors in various pathways in the brain. Atypical antipsychotics also enhance the effectiveness of serotonin.

Clinical Use. Table 21-8 lists the most frequently prescribed antipsychotic drugs. The chemical classes of the conventional, "typical" antipsychotic drugs are distinguished by the extent, type, and severity of side effects produced. Their overall clinical efficacy at equivalent doses is similar.

Table 21-8	Atypical Antipsychotic and Typical Antipsychotic Drugs				
GENERIC NAME (TRADE NAME)	THERAPEUTIC EQUIVALENT (POTENCY, MG)	HALF-LIFE (HR)	USUAL ADULT DAILY DOSE: RANGE (MG)*†	PREPARATIONS	
Atypical Antipsychotic Drugs					
Clozapine (Clozaril)	50	8-12	100-900	PO	
Risperidone (Risperdal, Consta)	0.5	3-24	2-8	PO, L, L-A	
Olanzapine (Zyprexa, Zydis)	5	27	5-20	PO, ODT	
Quetiapine (Seroquel)	50-100	7	150-750	PO	
Ziprasidone (Geodon)	40	5	40-160	PO, IM,	
Aripiprazole (Abilify)	5	50-80	10-15	PO	

*Dose is for PO unless noted.
†Dose range varies by patient and should be individualized.

IM, Intramuscular injection; L, oral liquid, elixir, suspension, concentrate; L-A, long-acting injectable preparation, ODT, orally disintegrating tablets; PO, oral tablet, capsule; Sup, suppository.

Generic Name (Trade Name)	Therapeutic Equivalent (Potency, MG)	Half-Life (HR)	Usual Adult Daily Dose: Range (MG)*†	Preparations
Typical Antipsychotic Drugs				
Phenothiazines				
Chlorpromazine (Thorazine)	100	23-37	200-1000	PO, IM, L, Sup
Thioridazine (Mellaril)	100	24-36	200-800‡	PO, IM, L
Mesoridazine (Serentil)	50	24-42	75-300	PO, IM, L
Perphenazine (Trilafon)	10	9	8-32	PO, IM, L
Trifluoperazine (Stelazine)	5	24	5-20	PO, IM, L
Fluphenazine (Prolixin)	2	22	2-60	PO, IM, L, L-A
Fluphenazine decanoate (Prolixin D)	.25 cc/month	q2-3 weeks	12.5-50 q 2-4 weeks	L-A
Thioxanthene				
Thiothixene (Navane)	4	34	5-30	PO, L, IM
Butyrophenone				
Haloperidol (Haldol)	2	24	2-20*	PO, IM, L
Haloperidol decanoate (Haldol D)	50-300	3 weeks	50-300 q 3-4 weeks	L-A

Continued

‡Upper limit to avoid retinopathy.

Table 21-8	Atypical Antipsychotic and Typical Antipsychotic Drugs—cont'd			
GENERIC NAME (TRADE NAME)	THERAPEUTIC EQUIVALENT (POTENCY, MG)	HALF-LIFE (HR)	USUAL ADULT DAILY DOSE: RANGE (MG)*†	PREPARATIONS
Dibenzoxazepine				
Loxapine (Loxitane)	10	4	20-100	PO, IM, L
Dihydroindolone				
Molindone (Moban)	10	1.5	50-225	PO, L
Diphenylbutylpiperidine				
Pimozide (Orap)	2	55	2-6	PO

IM, Intramuscular injection; *L,* oral liquid, elixir, suspension, concentrate; *L-A,* long-acting injectable preparation, *ODT,* orally disintegrating tablets; *PO,* oral tablet, capsule; *Sup,* suppository.

The newer, atypical antipsychotic drugs have clinical effects superior to other classes of antipsychotics with minimal acute extrapyramidal side effects.

The major uses of antipsychotic drugs are to manage schizophrenia, organic brain syndrome with psychosis, the manic phase of manic-depressive illness, and severe depression with psychosis. They are also useful for patients with severe anxiety who abuse drugs or alcohol because the benzodiazepines are contraindicated for them.

Adverse Reactions and Nursing Considerations. The side effects of antipsychotic drugs are many and varied and demand much clinical attention from the nurse for optimal care. Some side effects are merely uncomfortable for the patient, and most are easily treated, but some are life threatening. Table 21-9 summarizes these side effects and nursing considerations.

Table 21-9	Side Effects and Nursing Considerations: Antipsychotic Drugs
SIDE EFFECTS	NURSING CARE AND TEACHING CONSIDERATIONS
Extrapyramidal symptoms (EPS)	General treatment principles: 1. Tolerance usually develops by third month. 2. Decrease dose of drug. 3. Add a drug to treat EPS, then taper before 3 months of antipsychotic administration. 4. Use a drug with a lower EPS profile. 5. Provide patient education and support.

Continued

Table 21-9	Side Effects and Nursing Considerations: Antipsychotic Drugs—cont'd
SIDE EFFECTS	**NURSING CARE AND TEACHING CONSIDERATIONS**
1. Acute dystonic reactions: oculogyric crisis, torticollis (wryneck)	Frightening, painful spasms of major muscle groups of neck, back, and eyes; more common in children and young males and with high-potency drugs. Medicate with drugs to treat EPS; have respiratory support available. Taper dose gradually when discontinuing antipsychotics to avoid withdrawal dyskinesia.
2. Akathisia	Patient cannot remain still; pacing, inner restlessness, and leg aches are relieved by movement. Rule out anxiety or agitation; medicate.
3. Parkinson's syndrome: akinesia, cogwheel rigidity, fine tremor	More common in males and elderly patients; tolerance may not develop. Medicate with amantadine, a dopamine agonist (DA); patient must have good renal function.
4. Tardive dyskinesia (TD)	Can occur after use (usually long use) of conventional antipsychotics; stereotyped involuntary movements: tongue protrusion, lip smacking, chewing, blinking, grimacing, choreiform movements of limbs and trunk, foot tapping. Assess patient often; consider changing to atypical antipsychotic drug.

Table 21-9	Side Effects and Nursing Considerations: Antipsychotic Drugs—cont'd
SIDE EFFECTS	**NURSING CARE AND TEACHING CONSIDERATIONS**
Neuroleptic malignant syndrome (NMS)	Potentially fatal, with fever, tachycardia, sweating, muscle rigidity, tremor, incontinence, stupor, leukocytosis, elevated creatinine phosphokinase, renal failure; more common with high-potency drugs and in dehydrated persons. Discontinue all drugs; provide supportive symptomatic care: hydration, renal dialysis, ventilation, and fever reduction as appropriate; can treat with dantrolene or bromocriptine; antipsychotic drugs can be cautiously reintroduced over time.
Seizures	Occur in approximately 1% of patients taking antipsychotics; clozapine has a 5% seizure rate in patients taking 600-900 mg/day; may need to discontinue clozapine.
Other side effects	
1. Agranulocytosis	*This is an emergency;* it develops abruptly, with fever, malaise, ulcerative sore throat, and leukopenia. High incidence (1%-2%) is associated with clozapine; must do weekly complete blood counts and prescribe only 1 week of drug at a time; discontinue drug immediately; patient may need reverse isolation and antibiotics.
2. Photosensitivity	Use sunscreen and sunglasses; cover body with clothing.
3. Anticholinergic effects	Symptoms include constipation, dry mouth, blurred vision, orthostatic hypotension, tachycardia, urinary retention, nasal congestion. Decrease dose; use alternate drug.
4. Sedation, weight gain	Decrease dose; change drug; keep patient active; reduce calories.

♩ NURSE **ALERT**

- The nurse should pay particular attention to the **extrapyramidal symptoms** (EPS), both short term and long term. The most common drugs to treat short-term EPS follow:
  1. Benztropine, 1 to 6 mg/day
  2. Trihexyphenidyl, 1 to 10 mg/day
  3. Diphenhydramine, 25 to 150 mg/day
- The most serious adverse effect of clozapine is **agranulocytosis,** which occurs in approximately 1% to 2% of patients.
- A potentially fatal adverse reaction to antipsychotic medication is **neuroleptic malignant syndrome** (NMS).

♩ NURSE **ALERT**

Guidelines for antipsychotic drug administration:
1. Individualized dosage requirements for antipsychotic drugs vary greatly.
2. After initial divided doses, patients can receive doses once a day.
3. Symptom improvement usually occurs in 2 or 3 days to 2 weeks. Optimal effects may take several months.
4. Some patients require a lifetime of continuous antipsychotic medication treatment.
5. Observation for tardive dyskinesia (long-term EPS) should be done about monthly during long-term treatment with conventional antipsychotics.
6. Good clinical care for patients taking clozapine includes weekly complete blood counts to monitor for decreased white cell count and clozapine prescriptions given for 1 week at a time.

Your Internet Connection

Psychopharmacology Resources
www.psychwatch.com/psychopharm_page.htm

Psychopharmacology Tips
www.dr-bob.org/tips

US Food and Drug Administration
www.fda.gov/cder/drug/infopage/lotronex/lotronex.htm

Virtual Drug Store
www.virtualdrugstore.com

■ PHYSICAL RESTRAINTS

Physical restraint includes the use of mechanical restraints, such as wrist or ankle cuffs and restraining sheets, and seclusion, which is confinement to a room from which the patient is unable to exit at will. In this era of sensitivity to civil liberties and individual rights, restraint should be used with great discretion.

Mechanical Restraints

Types of mechanical restraints are (1) camisoles (straitjackets), (2) wrist cuff restraints, (3) ankle cuff restraints, and (4) sheet restraints.

♩ NURSE **ALERT**

Prevention of behavior necessitating restraints is the most important nursing action. Restraint is always an intervention of last resort.

Indications for Restraint.

1. Violent behavior that is dangerous to the patient or others
2. Agitated behavior that cannot be controlled by medication

3. Threat to physical integrity related to the patient's refusal to rest or eat and drink
4. Patient's request for external behavioral controls, provided this is assessed to be therapeutically indicated

Table 22-1 presents nursing interventions for restrained patients.

Table 22-1	Nursing Interventions for a Secluded or Mechanically Restrained Patient	
PRINCIPLE	**RATIONALE**	**NURSING INTERVENTIONS**
Patient has a right to least restrictive treatment.	This is a constitutional right of all patients.	Identify precipitating events. Observe patient for agitated behavior. Attempt alternative interventions. Document patient behavior and nursing interventions.
Protect patient from physical injury.	An individual who is not in control of behavior is at risk of injury and needs external limits, safely applied.	Provide adequate staff resources to control patient. Be sure staff is trained to manage violent behavior. Plan the approach to patient. Use safe physical restraint techniques.
Provide a safe environment.	An individual who is not in control of behavior may have impaired judgment and may harm self accidentally or purposefully.	Observe patient constantly or very frequently, depending on condition. Remove dangerous objects from area.

Continued

Table 22-1	Nursing Interventions for a Secluded or Mechanically Restrained Patient—cont'd	
PRINCIPLE	**RATIONALE**	**NURSING INTERVENTIONS**
Maintain biological integrity.	Physically restrained patients are not able to attend to their own biological needs and are at risk for complications related to immobility.	Check vital signs. Bathe patient and provide skin care. Take patient to bathroom or provide bedpan or urinal. Regulate room temperature. Place patient in anatomical position. Pad restraints. Offer food and fluids. Release restraints at least every 2 hours.
Maintain dignity and self-esteem.	Loss of control and imposition of physical restraint may be embarrassing to patient.	Provide privacy. Explain situation to other patients without revealing confidential patient information. Maintain verbal contact with patient at regular intervals while awake. Assign consistent staff member of same sex to provide personal care. Involve patient in plans to terminate physical restraint. Wean patient from protected setting.

⚕ NURSE **ALERT**

Patients in any type of physical restraint are highly vulnerable and must be protected.

Seclusion

Seclusion is confinement in a room that the patient is unable to leave at will. Degrees of seclusion may range from confinement in a room with a closed but unlocked door to a locked room with a mattress without linens on the floor, limited opportunity for communication, and the patient dressed in a hospital gown or a heavy canvas coverall. The latter are minimally acceptable conditions for seclusion and are used only when essential for the protection of the patient or others.

Indications for Seclusion.
1. Control of violent behavior that is potentially dangerous to the patient or others and cannot be controlled by other, less restrictive interventions such as interpersonal contact or medications
2. Reduction of environmental stimuli, particularly if requested by the patient

Contraindications for Seclusion.
1. Need for observation for a medical problem
2. High suicide risk
3. Potential for intolerance of sensory deprivation
4. Punishment

Table 22-1 presents nursing interventions for secluded patients. Box 22-1 outlines the procedure for managing psychiatric emergencies.

■ ELECTROCONVULSIVE THERAPY

Electroconvulsive therapy (ECT) artificially induces a grand mal seizure by passing an electrical current through electrodes applied to one or both temples. The number of treatments given in a series varies according to the patient's initial problem and therapeutic response as assessed during treatment. The most common range for affective disorders is 6 to

BOX 22-1

Procedure for Managing Psychiatric Emergencies

1. Identify crisis leader.
2. Assemble crisis team.
3. Notify security officers if necessary.
4. Remove all other patients from area.
5. Obtain restraints if appropriate.
6. Devise a plan to manage crisis and inform team.
7. Assign securing of patient's limbs to crisis team members.
8. Explain necessity of intervention to patient and attempt to enlist cooperation.
9. Restrain patient when directed by crisis leader.
10. Administer medication if ordered.
11. Maintain calm, consistent approach to patient.
12. Review crisis management interventions with crisis team.
13. Process events with other patients and staff as appropriate.
14. Gradually reintegrate patient into milieu.

12 treatments, whereas many more may be given for a patient with schizophrenia. ECT is usually administered 2 to 3 times a week on alternate days, although it can be given more or less frequently.

Indications for ECT

1. Patients with major depressive illness who have not responded to antidepressant medication or who are unable to take medication
2. Patients with bipolar disorder who have not responded to medication
3. Acutely suicidal patients who have not received medication long enough to achieve a therapeutic effect

4. When the anticipated side effects of ECT are less than those associated with drug therapy, such as with elderly patients, for patients with heart block, and during pregnancy

Procedure for ECT

1. Provide patient and family education about the procedure.
2. Obtain informed consent.
3. Ensure NPO (nothing by mouth) status of the patient after midnight.
4. Ask the patient to remove jewelry, hairpins, eyeglasses, and hearing aids. Full dentures are removed; partial plates remain in place.
5. Dress the patient in loose, comfortable clothing.
6. Have the patient empty bladder.
7. Administer pretreatment medications.
8. Ensure necessary drugs and equipment are available and in working order (Box 22-2).
9. Assist with administration of ECT.
   - Reassure the patient.
   - The physician or anesthesiologist administers oxygen to prepare the patient for the period of apnea that results from the muscle relaxant.
   - Administer medications.
   - Position padded mouth gag to protect the patient's teeth.
   - Position electrodes. The shock is then given.
10. Monitor the patient during the recovery period.
    - Assist as needed with the administration of oxygen and suctioning.
    - Monitor vital signs.
    - After respiration is established, position the patient on side until conscious. Maintain a patent airway.
    - When the patient is responsive, provide orientation.
    - Ambulate with assistance, after checking for postural hypotension.

BOX 22-2

Equipment for Electroconvulsive Therapy (ECT)

- Treatment device and supplies, including electrode paste and gel, gauze pads, alcohol preps, saline, electroencephalogram (EEG) electrodes, and chart paper
- Monitoring equipment, including electrocardiogram (ECG) and ECG electrodes
- Blood pressure cuffs (2), peripheral nerve stimulator, and pulse oximeter
- Stethoscope
- Reflex hammer
- Intravenous and venipuncture supplies
- Bite blocks with individual containers
- Stretcher with firm mattress and side rails and capability to elevate head and feet
- Suction device
- Ventilation equipment, including tubing, masks, Ambu bags, oral airways, and intubation equipment with an oxygen delivery system capable of providing positive-pressure oxygen
- Emergency and other medications as recommended by anesthesia staff
- Miscellaneous medications not supplied by the anesthesia staff for medical management during ECT, such as labetalol, esmolol, glycopyrrolate, caffeine, curare, midazolam, diazepam, thiopental sodium (Pentothal), methohexital sodium (Brevital Sodium), and succinylcholine

- Allow the patient to sleep for a short time if desired.
- Provide a light meal.
- Involve in usual daily activities, providing orientation as needed.
- Offer prescribed analgesia for headache as necessary.

Table 22-2	Nursing Interventions for a Patient Receiving Electroconvulsive Therapy (ECT)	
PRINCIPLE	RATIONALE	NURSING INTERVENTIONS
Obtain informed participation in the procedure.	A patient who understands the treatment plan will be more cooperative and experience less stress than one who does not. An informed family is able to provide patient with emotional support.	Educate about ECT, including procedure and expected effects. Teach family about treatment. Encourage expression of feelings by patient and family. Reinforce teaching after each treatment.
Maintain biological integrity.	General anesthesia and an electrically induced seizure are physiological stressors and require supportive nursing care.	Check emergency equipment before procedure. Keep patient NPO several hours before treatment. Remove potentially harmful objects (e.g., jewelry, dentures). Check vital signs.

Continued

Table 22-2 summarizes nursing interventions for the patient receiving ECT.

■ PHOTOTHERAPY

Phototherapy, or light therapy, consists of exposing patients to artificial therapeutic lighting about 5 to 20 times brighter than indoor lighting. Patients usually sit with eyes open, about 3 feet away from and at eye level with broad-spectrum

Table 22-2	Nursing Interventions for a Patient Receiving Electroconvulsive Therapy (ECT)—cont'd	
PRINCIPLE	RATIONALE	NURSING INTERVENTIONS
Maintain patient's dignity and self-esteem.	Patients are usually fearful before the treatment. Amnesia and confusion may lead to fear of becoming insane. Patient will need assistance to function appropriately in the milieu.	Maintain patent airway. Position on side until reactive. Assist to ambulate. Offer analgesia or antiemetic as needed. Remain with patient and offer support before and during treatment. Maintain patient's privacy during and after treatment. Reorient patient. Assist family members and other patients to understand behavior related to amnesia and confusion.

fluorescent bulbs designed to produce the intensity and color composition of outdoor light. The timing and dosage of light therapy vary for each patient. The brighter the light, the more effective is the treatment per unit of time.

Treatment is rapid and can be effective. Most patients feel relief after 3 to 5 days and relapse when treatment is stopped. Patients do not appear to develop tolerance to phototherapy, but its long-term efficacy has not been fully evaluated.

Phototherapy has a 50% to 60% response rate in patients with well-documented nonpsychotic winter depression or seasonal affective disorder (SAD). Light therapy should be administered by a professional with experience and training.

■ SLEEP DEPRIVATION THERAPY

It has been reported that as many as 60% of depressed patients improve immediately after one night of total sleep deprivation. However, few randomized controlled clinical studies have been conducted on sleep deprivation, thus these reports should be considered with caution. Unfortunately, many patients who respond to this therapy become depressed again when they resume sleeping even as little as 2 hours a night.

■ TRANSCRANIAL MAGNETIC STIMULATION

Transcranial magnetic stimulation (TMS) is a noninvasive procedure in which a changing magnetic field is introduced into the brain in order to influence the brain's activity. The field is generated by passing a large electric current through a wire stimulation coil for a brief period of time. The insulated coil is placed on or close to a specific area of the patient's head, allowing the magnetic field to pass through the skull and into target areas of the brain. The most frequently cited indication for TMS is in the treatment of mood disorders.

■ VAGUS NERVE STIMULATION

Vagus nerve stimulation (VNS) is the newest of the somatic therapies currently under investigation. A recent multicenter study showing a 40% to 50% reduction in depressive symptoms using VNS validates its potential as a promising new somatic therapy in psychiatry.

VNS involves surgically implanting a small (pocket watch-sized) generator into the patient's chest. An electrode is threaded subcutaneously from the generator to the vagus nerve on the left side of the patient's neck. The end of the electrode is wrapped around the nerve. Once implanted, the generator is programmed via computer for the frequency and intensity of the stimulus.

At present VNS is approved only for clinical use in the treatment of epilepsy. The most compelling use of VNS in psychiatry is in the treatment of affective disorders, particularly depression.

■ ALTERNATIVE THERAPIES

Complementary and alternative medicine (CAM) is the term commonly used to describe a broad range of healing philosophies, approaches, and therapies that focus on the whole person, including biopsychosocial and spiritual aspects. CAM therapies are often used alone (often referred to as *alternative*), in combination with other CAM therapies, or in combination with other conventional therapies (sometimes referred to as *complementary*).

Some therapies are consistent with principles of Western medicine, whereas others involve healing systems with a different origin. Although some therapies are outside the realm of accepted Western medical practice, others are becoming established in mainstream health care.

The National Center of Complementary and Alternative Medicine has identified the major domains of complementary and alternative medicine. Table 22-3 lists the domain, defines it, and provides the related CAM therapy.

There are a few well-designed CAM research studies in psychiatric illness mental health. Ethical concerns about CAM therapies include issues of safety and effectiveness and the expertise and qualifications of the practitioner. Of equal importance is the communication between the CAM provider and the traditional health care provider. Box 22-3 provides information that health consumers should consider when deciding on a complementary or alternative therapy.

Depression

Depression is one of the most common conditions for which people use alternative therapies. A review of the most

Table 22-3	Major Domains of Complementary and Alternative Medicine	
DOMAIN	**DEFINITION**	**CAM THERAPY**
Alternative medical systems	Complete systems of theory and practice that have evolved independently of, and often prior to, the conventional biomedical approach	Traditional oriental medicine, Ayurveda, homeopathy, naturopathy
Mind-body interventions	Employ a variety of techniques designed to facilitate the mind's capacity to affect bodily function and symptoms	Meditation; hypnosis; prayer; art, music, and dance therapy
Biologically based therapies	Natural and biologically based practices, interventions, and products, many of which overlap with conventional medicine's use of dietary supplements	Herbal, special dietary, orthomolecular, and individual biological therapies
Manipulative and body-based methods	Methods based on manipulation and/or movement of the body	Chiropractic, massage and body work, reflexology
Energy therapies	Focus on either energy fields believed to originate within the body (biofields) or those emanating from other sources (electromagnetic fields)	Qi gong, Reiki, therapeutic touch, electromagnets

From US Department of Health and Human Services: *Expanding horizons of healthcare: five-year strategic plan, 2001-2005*, NCCAM (SuDoc HE 20.3002: H 78), Washington, DC, 2000, USDHHS. *CAM*, Complementary and alternative medicine.

BOX 22-3

Approaching Complementary and Alternative Therapies

- Ask a health care provider about the safety and effectiveness of the desired therapy or treatment. Information can also be found in current publications and on the website of the NCCAM at the National Institutes of Health
- Contact a state or local regulatory agency with authority over practitioners who practice the therapy or treatment being sought. CAM usually is not as regulated as the practice of conventional medicine, but licensing, accreditation, and regulatory laws are increasingly being implemented. Check to see if the practitioner is licensed to deliver the identified services.
- Talk with those who have had experience with this practitioner, both health care providers and other patients. Find out about the confidence and competence of the practitioner and whether there have been any complaints from patients.
- Talk with the practitioner in person. Ask about education, additional training, licenses, and certifications, both conventional and unconventional. Find out how open the practitioner is to communicating with patients about technical aspects of methods, possible side effects, and potential problems.
- Visit the practitioner's office, clinic, or hospital. Ask how many patients are typically seen in a day or week and how much time is spent with each patient. Look at the conditions of the office or clinic. The primary issue here is whether the service delivery adheres to regulated standards for medical safety and care.
- Find out what several practitioners charge for the same treatment to get a better idea about the appropriateness of costs. Regulatory agencies and professional associations may also provide cost information.

BOX **22-3**

Approaching Complementary and Alternative
Therapies—cont'd

- Most importantly, discuss all issues concerning
  therapies and treatments with your usual health care
  provider, whether a practitioner of conventional or
  alternative medicine. Competent health care
  management requires knowledge of both conventional
  and alternative therapies for the provider to have a
  complete picture of your treatment plan.

beneficial CAM therapies for depression finds that there is
evidence to support the use of exercise, herbal therapy,
acupuncture, and massage therapy.

Anxiety

Anxiety disorders are cited as one of the major reasons people
use CAM therapies. Anxiety disorders that have been inves-
tigated using CAM therapies include generalized anxiety
disorders, social and specific phobias, panic disorder,
obsessive-compulsive disorder, and posttraumatic stress
disorder. Evidence suggests that relaxation, therapeutic
touch, yoga, and herbal products can reduce anxiety.

Substance Use Disorders

One of the most widely researched CAM therapies for
addiction is acupuncture, and a number of chemical dependency programs in the United States use acupuncture as an
additional therapy. One study supports the use of yoga in
reducing drug use, and there are some small studies reporting
the efficacy of biofeedback for the treatment of addictions.

In summary, CAM therapies can have an important
impact on psychiatric nursing practice. They can be bene-

ficial, safe, cost-effective, and easily implemented throughout psychiatric and medical settings. Nurses should continue to follow the research literature to ensure that patients receive only those treatments with a strong evidence base.

 Your Internet Connection

Acupuncture.com
www.acupuncture.com

Alternative Medicine Center
www.healthy.net/clinic/therapy/index.html

National Center for Complementary and Alternative Medicine
http://nccam.nih.gov

Aguilera DC: *Crisis intervention: theory and methodology*, ed 8, St Louis, 1998, Mosby.

Amador X: *I'm not sick, I don't need help!* Peconinc, NY, 2000, VidaPress.

American Nurses Association: *Code for nurses with interpretive statements*, Kansas City, Mo, 1985, The Association.

American Nurses Association: *Nursing's social policy statement*, Kansas City, Mo, 1995, The Association.

American Nurses Association: *Scope and standards of psychiatric–mental health clinical nursing practice*, Washington, DC, 2000, The Association.

American Psychiatric Association: *Diagnostic and statistical manual of mental disorders*, ed 4, text revision (DSM-IV-TR), Washington, DC, 2000, The Association.

American Psychiatric Association: *Handbook of psychiatric measures*, Washington, DC, 2000, The Association.

Anthony WA: *Principles of psychiatric rehabilitation*, Baltimore, 1999, University Park Press.

Bandura A: *Self-efficacy: the exercise of control*, New York, 1997, Freeman.

Bazelon Center for Mental Health Law: *Psychiatric advance directive*, Washington, DC, 1998, The Center.

Beck A, et al: *Cognitive therapy of depression*, New York, 1979, Guilford Press.

Bracken B: *Handbook of self-concept*, New York, 1996, John Wiley & Sons.

Department of Health and Human Services Steering Committee on the Chronically Mentally Ill: *Toward a national plan for the chronically mentally ill*, Pub No ADM-81-1077, Washington, DC, 1981, US Government Printing Office.

Egan A, Arnold R: Grief and bereavement care, *Am J Nurs* 103:42, 2003.

Endicott J, Spitzer RL, Fleiss JL, Cohen J: The global assessment scale. A procedure for measuring overall severity of psychiatric disturbance, *Arch Gen Psychiatry* 33:766-771, 1976.

Ewing JA: Detecting alcoholism: the CAGE Questionnaire, *JAMA* 252:1905, 1984.

Freeman L, Lawlis G: *Mosby's complementary and alternative medicine: a research-based approach*, St Louis, 2003, Mosby.

Geldmacher S: *Contemporary diagnosis and management of Alzheimer's disease*, Newtown, Pa, 2003, Handbooks in Health Care.

Hardin SB: Catastrophic stress. In McBride AB, Austin JK, editors: *Psychiatric–mental health nursing*, Philadelphia, 1996, WB Saunders.

Holt J: How to help confused patients, *Am J Nurs* 93(8):32, 1993.

Institute of Medicine: *Reducing suicide: a national imperative*, Washington, DC, 2002, National Academies Press.

Joint Commission on Accreditation of Healthcare Organizations: *Preventing patient suicide*, Oakbrook Terrace, Ill, 2000, The Commission.

Joint Commission Resources: *Front line of defense: the role of nurses in preventing sentinel events*, Oakbrook Terrace, Ill, 2001, The Commission.

Kay J, Tasman A, editors: *Psychiatry: behavioral science and clinical essentials*, Philadelphia, 2000, WB Saunders.

Koenig H, McCullogh M, Larson D: *Handbook of religion and health*, Oxford, 2001, Oxford University Press.

Linehan M: *Skills training manual for treating borderline personality disorder*, New York, 1993, Guilford Press.

Luborsky L: The global assessment scale: a procedure for measuring overall severity of psychiatric disturbance, *Arch Gen Psychiatry* 7:407-417, 1962.

Manderscheid R, Henderson M, editors: *Mental health—United States, 2003*, Washington, DC, 2004, Department of Health and Human Services, Center for Mental Health Services.

Miracle TS, Miracle AW, Baumeister RF: *Human sexuality: meeting your basic needs*, Upper Saddle River, NJ, 2003, Prentice Hall.

Monat A, Lazarus R: *Stress and coping*, New York, 1991, Columbia University Press.

Mrazek P, Haggerty R: *Reducing risks for mental disorders*, Washington, DC, 1994, National Academy Press.

Mruk C: *Self-esteem: research, theory and practice*, New York, 1999, Springer.

Mueser KT, et al: Illness management and recovery: a review of the research, *Psychiatr Serv* 53:1272, 2002.

Murray C, Lopez A: *The global burden of disease: a comprehensive assessment of mortality and disability from disease, injuries, and risk factors in 1990 and projected to 2020*, Cambridge, Mass, 1996, Harvard University Press.

Nathan P, Gorman J: *A guide to treatments that work*, ed 2, New York, 2002, Oxford University Press.

New Freedom Commission on Mental Health: *Achieving the promise: transforming mental health care in America*, DHHS Pub No SMA-03-3832, Rockville, Md, 2003, Department of Health and Human Services.

Nolte J: *The human brain: an introduction to its functional anatomy*, ed 5, St Louis, 2002, Mosby.

Norbeck J et al: Social support needs of family caregivers of psychiatric patients from three age groups, *Nurs Res* 40:208, 1991.

North American Nursing Diagnosis Association: *NANDA nursing diagnoses: definitions and classification 2005-2006*, Philadelphia, 2003, NANDA.

Pardes H: The Report of the National Advisory Mental Health Council: *Am J Psychiatry* 150:1447, 1993.

Robinson D: *The mental status exam explained,* New York, 2002, Rapid Psychler Press.

Schatzberg A, Nemeroff C: *Textbook of psychopharmacology,* ed 3, Washington, DC, 2004, AP Publishing.

Skinner HA: The Drug Abuse Screening Test, *Addict Behav* 7(4):363, 1982.

Stuart G, Laraia M: *Principles and practice of psychiatric nursing,* ed 8, St Louis, 2005, Mosby.

Stuart G: Recent changes and current issues in psychiatric nursing. In McCloskey J, editor: *Current issues in nursing,* St Louis, 2001, Mosby.

Substance Abuse and Mental Health Services Administration: *Enhancing motivation for change in substance abuse treatment, Treatment Improvement Protocol Series #35,* Rockville, Md, 1999, Department of Health and Human Services.

Sundeen S, et al: *Nurse-client interaction: implementing the nursing process,* ed 6, St Louis, 1998, Mosby.

Taylor C, Altman T: Priorities in prevention research for eating disorders, *Psychopharm Bull* 33(3):413, 1997.

Thibodeau GA, Patton KT: *The human body in health and disease,* ed 4, 2005, Mosby.

Torrey EF: *Surviving schizophrenia,* ed 4, New York, 2001, Harper Collins.

US Department of Health and Human Services: *Expanding horizons of healthcare: five-year strategic plan, 2001-2005,* NCCAM (SuDoc HE 20.3002: H 78), Washington, DC, 2000, Department of Health and Human Services.

US Department of Health and Human Services: *Healthy people 2010,* Washington, DC, 2000, Department of Health and Human Services.

US Department of Health and Human Services: *Mental health: a report of the Surgeon General,* Rockville, Md, 1999, National Institute of Mental Health.

US Department of Health and Human Services: *Mental health: culture, race and ethnicity*, Rockville, Md, 2001, Office of the Surgeon General.

US Department of Health and Human Services: *Training manual for mental health and human service workers in major disasters*, ed 2, Washington, DC, 2000, US Government Printing Office.

US Department of Health and Human Services: *National strategy for suicide prevention: goals and objectives for action*, Rockville, Md, 2001, Department of Health and Human Services.

US Preventive Services Task Force: Screening for depression: recommendations and rationale, *Am J Nurs* 102:77, 2002.

US Public Health Service: *Surgeon General's call to action to prevent suicide*, Washington, DC, 1999, US Public Health Service.

Vaillant G: *The wisdom of the ego*, Cambridge, Mass, 1993, Harvard University Press.

Wells A: *Cognitive therapy of anxiety disorders: a practice manual and conceptual guide*, New York, 1997, John Wiley.

Wiger D, Huntley D: *Essentials of interviewing*, New York, 2002, John Wiley & Sons.

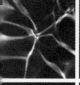

INDEX

Page numbers followed by "f" denote figures, "t"
denote tables, and "b" denote boxes.

450

NANDA Diagnoses

Activity intolerance
Activity intolerance, Risk for
Adjustment, Impaired
Airway clearance, Ineffective
Allergy response, Latex
Allergy response, Risk for latex
Anxiety
Anxiety, Death
Aspiration, Risk for
Attachment, Risk for impaired parent/infant/child
Autonomic dysreflexia
Autonomic dysreflexia, Risk for
Body image, Disturbed
Body temperature, Risk for imbalanced
Bowel incontinence
Breastfeeding, Effective
Breastfeeding, Ineffective
Breastfeeding, Interrupted
Breathing pattern, Ineffective
Cardiac output, Decreased
Caregiver role strain
Caregiver role strain, Risk for
Comfort, Impaired
Communication, Impaired verbal
Conflict, Decisional
Conflict, Parental role
Confusion, Acute
Confusion, Chronic
Constipation
Constipation, Perceived
Constipation, Risk for
Coping, Ineffective
Coping, Ineffective community
Coping, Readiness for enhanced community
Coping, Defensive
Coping, Compromised family
Coping, Disabled family
Coping, Readiness for enhanced family
Denial, Ineffective
Dentition, Impaired
Development, Risk for delayed
Diarrhea

Disuse syndrome, Risk for
Diversional activity, Deficient
Energy field, Disturbed
Environmental interpretation syndrome, Impaired
Failure to thrive, Adult
Falls, Risk for
Family processes: alcoholism, Dysfunctional
Family processes, Interrupted
Fatigue
Fear
Fluid volume, Deficient
Fluid volume, Excess
Fluid volume, Risk for deficient
Fluid volume, Risk for imbalanced
Gas exchange, Impaired
Grieving
Grieving, Anticipatory
Grieving, Dysfunctional
Grieving, Risk for dysfunctional
Growth and development, Delayed
Growth, Risk for disproportionate
Health maintenance, Ineffective
Health-seeking behaviors
Home maintenance, Impaired
Hopelessness
Hyperthermia
Hypothermia
Identity, Disturbed personal
Incontinence, Functional urinary
Incontinence, Reflex urinary
Incontinence, Stress urinary
Incontinence, Total urinary
Incontinence, Urge urinary
Incontinence, Risk for urge urinary
Infant behavior, Disorganized
Infant behavior, Risk for disorganized
Infant behavior, Readiness for enhanced organized
Infant feeding pattern, Ineffective
Infection, Risk for
Injury, Risk for
Injury, Risk for perioperative-positioning